Morning
Strength
Workouts

Morning *Strength* Workouts

Annette Lang

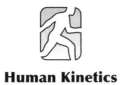

Human Kinetics

Library of Congress Cataloging-in-Publication Data

Lang, Annette, 1959-
  Morning strength workouts / Annette Lang.
      p. cm.
  Includes index.
  ISBN-13: 978-0-7360-6064-6 (soft cover)
  ISBN-10: 0-7360-6064-2 (soft cover)
  1. Exercise. 2. Weight training. 3. Physical fitness. I. Title.
  RA781.L36 2007
  613.7'1--dc22   2006023710

ISBN-10: 0-7360-6064-2
ISBN-13: 978-0-7360-6064-6

Acquisitions Editor: Martin Barnard; **Developmental Editor:** Amanda M. Eastin; **Assistant Editor:** Christine Horger; **Copyeditor:** Elizabeth Foz; **Proofreader:** Erin Cler; **Indexers:** Robert and Cynthia Swanson; **Permission Manager:** Carly Breeding; **Graphic Designer:** Bob Reuther; **Graphic Artist:** Kim McFarland; **Photo Managers:** Joe Jovanovich and Brenda Williams; **Cover Designer:** Keith Blomberg; **Photographer (cover):** © Angela Wyant/Getty Images; **Photographer (interior):** Brenda Williams; **Art Manager:** Kelly Hendren; **Illustrator:** Argosy; **Printer:** Sheridan Books

Human Kinetics books are available at special discounts for bulk purchase. Special editions or book excerpts can also be created to specification. For details, contact the Special Sales Manager at Human Kinetics.

Printed in the United States of America   10   9   8   7   6   5   4   3   2   1

Human Kinetics
Web site: www.HumanKinetics.com

United States: Human Kinetics
P.O. Box 5076
Champaign, IL 61825-5076
800-747-4457
e-mail: humank@hkusa.com

Canada: Human Kinetics
475 Devonshire Road Unit 100
Windsor, ON N8Y 2L5
800-465-7301 (in Canada only)
e-mail: orders@hkcanada.com

Europe: Human Kinetics
107 Bradford Road
Stanningley
Leeds LS28 6AT, United Kingdom
+44 (0) 113 255 5665
e-mail: hk@hkeurope.com

Australia: Human Kinetics
57A Price Avenue
Lower Mitcham, South Australia 5062
08 8372 0999
e-mail: liaw@hkaustralia.com

New Zealand: Human Kinetics
Division of Sports Distributors NZ Ltd.
P.O. Box 300 226 Albany
North Shore City
Auckland
0064 9 448 1207
e-mail: info@humankinetics.co.nz

This book is dedicated to Scott.
You can share my vegetable dumplings anytime!

part one   *AM Readiness*   1

part two   *Workouts for Every Schedule*   81

Contents

Preface

Mornings can be hectic, and your time is valuable. If you're looking for efficient, effective workouts that will fit into your busy morning schedule and give you the specific results you want, *Morning Strength Workouts* is the book for you. Since I entered the fitness industry in 1983, I've helped thousands of people reach their goals through their workouts. This book covers everything you need to plan and customize your workout routine by yourself, providing many workout options based on the amount of time you have available and your specific strength training goals. It includes all the components of a fitness program that a personal trainer would go over with you in order to design something that really works for your lifestyle and your goals. In addition, this book provides workout support in areas such as nutrition and hydration, rest needs, choosing the right equipment to meet your goals, and creating a workout space that will enhance your morning routine.

The book is divided into three parts. Part I helps you lay the groundwork for your program with information on how to optimize all the different aspects of your morning workout. Chapter 1 details the ins and outs of a lifestyle that gives you ample energy for your routines. It gives you advice on getting enough sleep, recommendations on nutrition and hydration (some of which might surprise you), and some ways to motivate yourself on those occasional mornings when you seem to have trouble getting going. This chapter will provide you with the knowledge and insight you need to make smart choices that will help you be ready for your morning routines—and have plenty of energy for the entire day.

Chapter 2 covers your options for where you do your morning workouts—at home, at the gym, or even outdoors. Whether you work out exclusively at home or also belong to a gym, setting up a workout space where you live can save valuable time during your busy mornings. This chapter shows you how to create a space that will make your workout comfortable and efficient. It covers topics from the energizing benefits of fresh air to where to store your equipment. It includes a list of the necessary equipment for setting up a home gym and instructions on how to make simple changes to your routine if needed. It also explains how you can get a great workout at a local playground and offers numerous tips on how to get the most out of your gym workout.

Should you use cables, free weights, machines, or your own body weight to challenge your muscles? What are the differences between these options, and how do they influence your choice of workout? Chapter 3 covers the various kinds of equipment available for your morning strength workouts. It explains the pros and cons of each type and how to use them safely and effectively. You'll learn how to substitute one piece of equipment for another if what you need is unavailable so that you can always get a great workout.

Chapter 4 will help you prepare your body for your morning workout using integrated training techniques, something that sets this book apart from others on the market. It discusses proper alignment and why good posture is so important. It also explains joint and muscle integrity and shows you how to get and keep your joints in proper balance. Stretches, muscle releases, and corrective exercises are given to help your body function at its best. Stretches lengthen muscles in order to allow a healthy range of motion around your joints, which is an important consideration in the morning after you've been sleeping all night. Muscle releases have the same purpose. Corrective exercises are designed to get your muscles to fire in the correct sequence, strengthening weak muscles so that other parts of your body don't get strained compensating for them. Exercising in the morning also requires a thorough and effective warm-up, and this chapter gives you four options that are very different from the traditional warm-ups you've probably been doing until now. Traditional warm-ups are done on cardiovascular machines—many times, this means peddling too slowly and with poor posture on a stationary bicycle. The integrated warm-ups in chapter 4 get all the parts of your body working together to improve your coordination, which will make your weightlifting efforts more efficient. They really get your blood flowing, giving you the energy you need for your early-morning routines. They also ensure that you get a safe workout, warming up your joints and challenging them through different ranges of motion to prepare you for all the exercises of your comprehensive strength program.

Chapter 5 gives you the essential information you need to determine your workout goals and reach them without wasted time or effort. So many people don't succeed in their strength training programs because they forget to have a plan. When you're exercising in the morning, time is of the essence. In order to be sure you are on the path to reach your goals, you need to understand exactly what to do to get the specific results you want. This chapter will help you customize the workouts in the book by providing information on how much weight you should lift and how intensely you should work depending on your goals. You will gain a clear understanding of how to make simple changes to make a workout more or less challenging and incorporate important but often neglected components of fitness, such as balance.

Part II of the book focuses on the workouts themselves. Chapters 6 through 9 are where you'll find the actual workouts, with lots of choices for your morning routines. They are grouped by how long the workouts take—chapter 6 lists 20-minute routines, chapter 7 lists 30-minute routines, chapter 8 lists 45-minute routines, and chapter 9 lists 60-minute routines. Each chapter contains five workouts—one each for strength, size, endurance, power, and general health and fitness. You can choose the type of workout based on your goals as discussed in chapter 5, and you can choose the length of the workout based on how much time you have and how you are feeling that morning.

Part III gives detailed descriptions of all of the individual exercises that make up the workouts in part II. Chapter 10 presents upper-body exercises, chapter 11 presents exercises for your core, and chapter 12 presents lower-body exercises.

In these chapters, you will also find quite a few exercises that work muscles in the upper and lower body at the same time. Many of the exercises have several versions that use different kinds of equipment. For example, there are multiple variations of a row that employ dumbbells, tubing, a cable, or a machine. Which one you pick will depend on your individual goals and what you have available. Seeing the exercises done with a different piece of equipment makes it easy for you to substitute one for another when you need to modify a workout. In addition to clear explanations of each exercise, these chapters include photographs that illustrate proper technique at every step of the way so you can make sure you are using good form.

Whether you are an experienced exerciser looking for new ideas for your morning routines or are new to morning exercise and want guidance on how to set up your strength routines to meet your goals, this book provides workouts to fit your needs. If you're looking for one reference to help you develop your own comprehensive strength training program and keep you moving efficiently in the morning, then *Morning Strength Workouts* will be an invaluable addition to your workout bag.

Acknowledgments

Working in fitness is the only real job I have ever had. Although I always knew I wanted to work in this field, it took quite a few years of tweaking to get to where I am now, and there are many people to thank.

My parents instilled a strong work ethic in me, and even though they haven't always understood exactly what I "do" in fitness, they have always been supportive and impressed by my stories and efforts. My brother and sisters are the best!

Joe Cirulli, Jan, and all the folks at the Gainesville Health and Fitness Center helped me realize that *sales* is not a dirty word but rather an opportunity to talk to people and help them find the motivation to make positive changes in their health and fitness. Bob Esquerre, who hired me at Equinox Fitness Club in New York City, was instrumental in my path to becoming an educator of personal trainers. I owe him a huge thank you. I also worked with Reebok University, which enabled me to meet wonderful people and learn a great deal about serving fitness professionals, and, ultimately, the consumer. I thank Stephanie Montgomery for supporting me in developing the personal training education programs for Reebok University. It was great to meet Gray Cook, who taught me so much about evaluating people's movements and enriched my skills as a teacher and trainer.

I appreciate all the managers, owners, and personal trainers I have met through the years who have helped me become a better educator. I also thank my clients—people who want to improve their fitness level and thereby enhance other aspects of their lives.

My friends in Brooklyn are a continual reminder of why I'm glad I'm not a fitness zealot. I like to have fun, and I don't live for fitness. I use and appreciate movement and exercise to help me with the rest of my life, not the reverse. My desire is simply to help people move more and feel better about themselves.

Finally, I would like to thank Human Kinetics for giving me this opportunity to further my efforts by publishing this book. Thanks to Sara Kooperman for referring them to me. Let's move more.

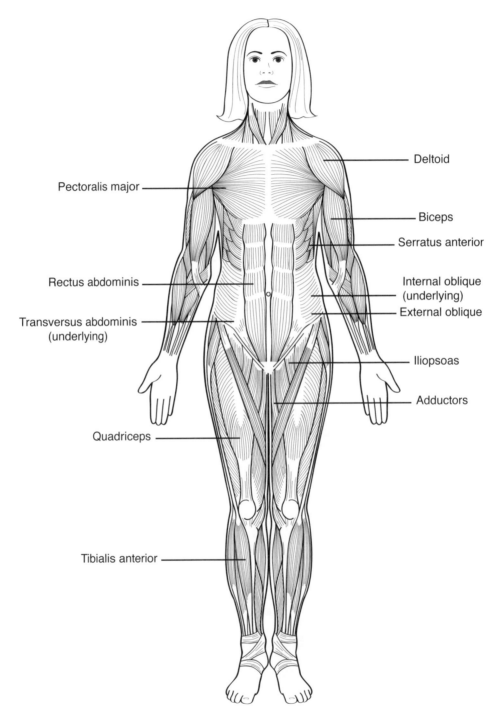

Deltoid

Pectoralis major

Biceps

Serratus anterior

Rectus abdominis

Internal oblique
(underlying)

External oblique

Transversus abdominis
(underlying)

Iliopsoas

Adductors

Quadriceps

Tibialis anterior

Reprinted, by permission, from S. Cole, 2003, *Athletic abs* (Champaign, IL: Human Kinetics), 24.

Guide to Muscles

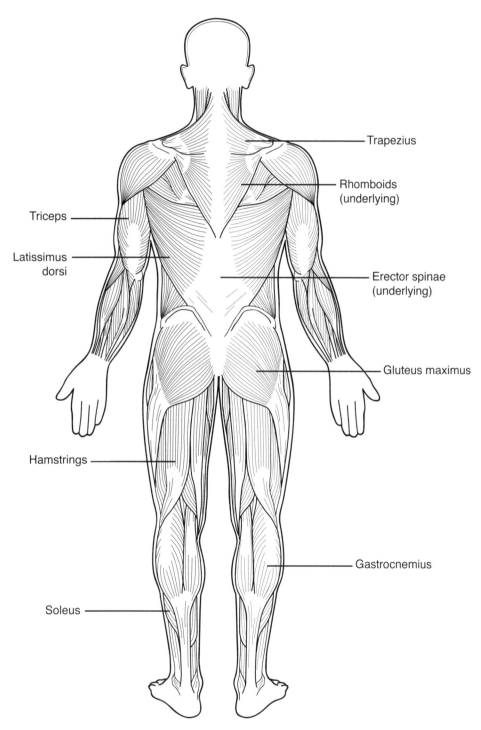

Trapezius

Rhomboids
(underlying)

Triceps

Latissimus
dorsi

Erector spinae
(underlying)

Gluteus maximus

Hamstrings

Gastrocnemius

Soleus

Reprinted, by permission, from S. Cole, 2003, *Athletic abs* (Champaign, IL: Human Kinetics), 24.

AM Readiness

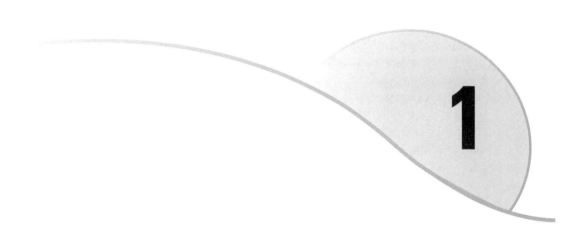

Energy to Begin Your Day

As a morning exerciser, you may have gone through many different phases of trying to get yourself motivated until you finally found what worked for you so that it was no longer difficult to be consistent with your routines. Or perhaps you are just getting started as a morning exerciser. Either way, this book will help you develop an effective, efficient, and fun program.

The benefits of regular exercise are well documented. We get these benefits—including lower blood pressure, higher HDL (good cholesterol) and lower LDL (bad cholesterol), increased metabolism, better-regulated blood sugar levels, improved mental capacity and mood, stronger joints, and greater bone density—regardless of what time of day we exercise.

So why are you more successful exercising in the morning than someone else? You probably know other people who are exactly the opposite way. They find they are better suited to exercising later in the day and would never consider getting up early to do it. The pattern of your energy levels throughout the day is partly due to your individual biological makeup. If you enjoy working out early in the day, it's likely that you consider yourself a morning person as opposed to a night owl. Some of the characteristics of a morning person are that you wake up fairly easily and do not always rely on an alarm clock. You have plenty of energy in the morning and feel alert at work, much to the annoyance of your night-owl coworkers! You work on challenging projects in the morning rather than later in the day, when you tend to feel more fatigued and less able to concentrate. This makeup contributes to making you a successful morning exerciser.

By making a deliberate decision to do something positive for yourself immediately after waking up, you improve your self-esteem, self-image, and your subconscious opinion of yourself. (Remember, your subconscious does not recognize what is true or untrue in an abstract sense, only what you reinforce by your thoughts and, especially, your actions.) Committing to a morning exercise program demonstrates that you are in control and gives you a feeling of accomplishment before you even get to work. This positive attitude tends to snowball during the day, giving you extra motivation to work on challenging projects. The rest of the day appears less overwhelming when you begin it with a success.

This chapter covers some important factors to enhance the success of your morning workout program. The main issues covered here are sleep, nutrition and hydration, and stress and motivation. The importance of getting enough sleep is the first topic, since by definition, early-morning workouts involve getting up on time in the morning. Everyone knows it's probably a good idea to get enough sleep, but what exactly does that mean? It is not just the actual act of sleeping that is important to the success of your workouts. As we'll explore, the quality as well as quantity of your sleep is affected by the interaction of many lifestyle factors during the day.

Proper nutrition is also discussed, both in general and more specifically in terms of how it affects exercising in the morning. What are the best choices for food and drinks, and what should you keep in mind before, during, and after your workout? When you eat in a healthy manner and drink enough water, you feel a general sense of well-being, and you perform better during your morning workouts as well as during the workday and any other activities you participate in.

This chapter also discusses motivation and stress. How can exercising in the morning help you better deal with stress during the rest of the day? What about acute stressors like a major life change or an unusually challenging or upsetting situation? Getting through these stressful times without skipping workouts or stopping them altogether can be tough, but it's important. If you understand the benefits of exercise, especially morning exercise, you will find the motivation to get through the everyday stressors as well as the really big ones that are also a part of life.

Sleep and Daily Habits

Sleep is crucially important to the human body, although it's easy to take for granted. After all, you don't have to think about it; it just happens naturally—or does it? If you've lost sight of the importance of sleep, just think of the times you've had trouble sleeping, and you will relish the thought of a good night's sleep again!

Think of sleep as the time your body gets to rest, repair, and grow. During the day, your body is so busy doing all the things you're asking it to do at any given moment that it doesn't have time to catch up, recover, and get stronger. Your immune system is constantly fighting germs, infection, and toxins such as pollution, exhaust, and many other things you encounter through your day. You take in viruses and bacteria by touching objects, breathing in the air around you, and eating food that is sometimes contaminated because of improper preparation or storage. All these stressors cumulatively trigger your body's natural *fight-or-flight* response, meaning it prepares itself to combat the stressful components. This causes your heart rate and blood pressure to increase. To prepare your body to react to the stress, it stimulates the secretion of stress hormones such as cortisol, causing cholesterol to flow more easily through your bloodstream. This process makes it easier for fatty deposits to get stuck on your artery walls, which increases your risk of heart disease and other health problems. External stress can wear down your cells and make them more susceptible to inflammation, which is also thought to be associated with heart disease and other potentially debilitating conditions. That's a lot of stress on your body, and it's coming from things that you don't even normally pay attention to during the day! More likely, you're aware of more noticeable things that can wear you down, such as your work, family, or financial responsibilities. The stress we encounter these days is chronic, making it difficult for your body to recuperate. This is where sleep comes in. Sleep is the time when your body can work toward repairing any damage that has happened and enhance its protective capabilities that help you stay well. After a good night's sleep, your body is ready to begin the daily cycle again.

There are other benefits of getting enough sleep that last throughout the day. Being well rested makes it easier to resist having several coffee drinks or sweet snacks in order to artificially elevate your energy. It means you have enough energy after work to do something besides spend a few hours sitting in front of the television or computer. Instead, you'll feel motivated both physically and mentally to do something a little more active, like taking a walk or going out to the movies. Getting enough sleep also means you feel a good kind of tired toward the very end of your day, and you look forward to going to sleep at a reasonable time.

When you work out in the morning, you need to have enough good-quality sleep so that your exercise routine is not compromised because you're feeling tired or run down. Working out in the morning means you don't have the extra time to prepare and get yourself feeling "up"; it's now or never! To get the most out of your program, you need to determine what helps you get enough good-quality sleep.

How much sleep does a person need to be able to function efficiently? You've probably heard throughout your life that you should get seven or eight hours, which is the across-the-board average recommendation. In fact, you might do just fine with six hours of sleep, or you might be someone who really needs more like eight to nine hours. You probably have noticed that on some mornings you get up quite easily, feeling refreshed. Then there are in-between mornings when you can get up, work out, and function fairly well. Finally, there are those times when you've gotten less than a certain amount of sleep and you're likely to skip your morning workout and feel lethargic all day. So, if you haven't already taken note of how much you slept the nights before these three types of mornings, how do you determine the right amount of sleep for you? One way to judge how well rested you are is whether you need an alarm clock to wake up in the morning. If you get enough sleep, you probably don't need one and can wake up naturally. Conversely, you can gauge whether you're sleep deprived by noticing how quickly you fall asleep when sitting still. If you fall asleep as soon as you sit down and stop moving—for example, on a train or in a car (when someone else is driving!)—then you are probably sleep deprived.

Sleep is intertwined with many other components of your life, and taking a close look at the other factors that influence your energy levels can help you analyze which habits benefit your sleep and your energy and which ones could use a change. This will help you get the most out of your early-morning workouts. Do this by keeping track of these components for two to four weeks and then seeing what patterns you can find. (There is a sample log in chapter 5 that shows you a good way to organize your observations.) Record the time you go to sleep and the time you get up. Note the day of the week. Write down how you feel and what your energy level is—high, moderate, low, or very low—at four points during the day: when you get up, at noon, at 3 p.m., and at 8 p.m. Also record other aspects of your lifestyle on a daily basis, such as eating; drinking; stressors and stress levels; and social, leisure, and fitness activities.

When you look over your notes, you'll begin to see how your sleep, daily habits, and energy during different times of the day are interrelated. For example, if you sometimes feel low-energy in the middle of the afternoon and have always assumed this was because you didn't get enough sleep the night before, you might realize that this only happens when you skip lunch. You might also notice that on many of those days you eat a chocolate bar to try to boost your energy. In this scenario, your low energy is not at all the result of getting inadequate sleep, but rather of skipping lunch, which lowers your blood sugar. This in turn leads to poor snack choices in the afternoon. Keeping track of your daily lifestyle choices can help you identify negative cycles like this one, as well as other potential problem areas. If you tweak your schedule and habits in response, you'll be more energetic and effective for your morning workouts and your entire day. After tracking and analyzing your habits over several weeks, you will find what works best for you.

Sometimes, despite our best efforts, we just can't fall asleep at night. Luckily, there are some things you can do to get both your body and your mind to slow down toward the end of the day, preparing you for a satisfying night of sleep.

- **Choose food and drink carefully.** If you eat a big meal right before you go to sleep, your stomach will be too full, making you feel uncomfortable and making it more difficult to fall asleep. Going to bed with a full stomach also compromises the quality of your sleep as your body must work to digest the food. Caffeine and alcohol consumption can also affect the quality of your sleep. If you have trouble falling asleep, look back through your notes and you might see that you tend to drink coffee (or another drink that has caffeine, like cola or black tea) late in the afternoon or after dinner. If this is the case, switching to decaffeinated drinks after lunchtime should help. Some herbal teas without caffeine, such as chamomile, can help you relax at bedtime. Many people also like warm milk, because it is soothing to the stomach and contains tryptophan, an amino acid that makes us feel drowsy. Some people feel they can fall asleep more easily if they have a drink at night. Alcohol *can* make it easier to fall asleep, but it can also make you wake up in the middle of the night after its effects wear off, and then it's harder to fall asleep again. Waking up in the middle of the night disturbs your body's natural sleep rhythms, and you won't feel refreshed in the morning. Again, keeping track of these habits will give you insight into what works best for you.

• **Avoid stressors.** Avoid watching potentially overstimulating television shows or movies right before you go to bed. These can get your mind stirred up and elevate your blood pressure and heart rate. By the same token, working on a business project that is stressful to you might not be the best way to get ready for sleep. Neither is paying bills! Do not exercise strenuously before bed, because that will rev up your metabolism rather than help you relax. Instead, you can try techniques such as deep breathing, meditation, or some of the stretches in chapter 4 to wind down.

• **Soothe your senses.** You might find that a warm shower or bath (with or without bath salts or oils) helps you relax at the end of the day. Experiment with some incense or candles to see if that makes you feel calm and sleepy. Some people like to use lavender oil or other essential oils in a scent diffuser to provide some soothing aromatherapy.

• **Create a calming atmosphere.** The room you sleep in can affect the quality of your night. Try to reserve your bedroom for sleeping and not use it for watching television or working. If your office is in your bedroom, at night you'll probably be tempted to check your e-mail one more time before going to bed. Mentally, it is relaxing to be able to associate this one room with quiet and sleep time instead of with stressful work. If light from the street comes in your windows, getting some dark drapes or curtains for the room might help you as well. These drapes should be easy to pull open so that you can still get natural light in the mornings. Adjusting your sleep habits to the natural light and dark of day and night will help you get up more easily for your morning workout.

The noise level around you can also affect the quality of your sleep. Some people need some background noise, such as sounds from the television or radio, to fall asleep. You might find it relaxing, but then it can wake you up later in the night. If you can set your television or radio to automatically shut off in 60 minutes, it might help you to fall asleep and stay asleep through the night. Another tip is to find some soothing music to play instead of traditional radio stations. Recordings of gentle ocean surf and other pleasing natural sounds have become very popular as well.

When things just don't go as planned and for some reason you don't get a good night's sleep, no need to fret. The workouts in chapters 6 through 9 are designed so that you can adjust your routine the next morning. If you get up later than you intended and you had planned to do a 60-minute workout for strength, you can do the 30- or 45-minute routine instead. Or, let's say you wanted to really work hard, but because you didn't sleep well during the night you don't have the energy for a challenging routine. You can change the focus of the workout by picking one for endurance instead of strength, which means that you will use less weight and not have to work so hard. You could also just choose a routine for general fitness instead of one of the more focused routines. The workouts for general fitness recommend that you not work to failure, meaning that you should stop before you reach the point of being unable to continue—this makes them a little less demanding. You can consider them "maintenance" routines that don't make you work as hard but still help you keep up your fitness level and strength. The flexibility that the routines in this book offer will allow you to achieve the most important thing, which is staying consistent with your program.

Nutrition and Hydration

Nutrition is your fuel. If you give your body the best fuel in the amounts that it needs, it will run well. Think of your body in the same way you think of a car. If you put the highest quality of gasoline into your car and keep it tuned up as required, it will run at its best.

What is your diet? I use the word *diet* to mean "eating habits," not a temporary plan designed to help you lose weight. There are many different theories about the best way to eat, the best kinds of food to eat, and how much of a given type of food you need. Numerous health and medical associations, including the American Heart Association and the U.S. Food and Drug Administration, recommend that eating plans be based on a proportion of approximately 60 percent carbohydrate, 30 percent fat (of which no more than a third—that is, 10 percent of total calories—should be saturated), and 10 percent protein. So if you count your calories and determine that you eat approximately 2,000 calories a day, for example, you should aim to get 1,200 (60 percent) of those calories from carbohydrate; no more than 600 calories (30 percent) from fat, of which no more than 200 calories (10 percent of overall calories) would be from saturated fat and the rest would be from unsaturated fat; and 200 calories (10 percent) from protein.

Carbohydrate, fat, and protein are called *macronutrients*. Macronutrients give your body the energy necessary to maintain normal functions, whether you are sedentary or active. This means your bones, your brain, and all of your other organs get the fuel and building materials they need in order to keep you alive and functional. You might think that the recommended 30 percent of total calories from fat is a high percentage. In fact, U.S. organizations have been struggling to get the average American to reduce their fat intake to that level. Diets with less than 30 percent of calories from fat do contribute to better health, especially if they are relatively high in unsaturated fats. Diets with extremely low levels of fat have been shown to help slow the progress of heart disease, but they are very difficult to sustain.

Active people need more calories than less active people, but experts debate whether active individuals need more of *certain nutrients* than less active individuals. As far as the proportions of carbohydrate, fat, and protein are concerned, there is not much solid evidence that a much higher percentage of any is necessary. A marathon runner might crave extra carbohydrate, since that is the body's preferred fuel source for sustained cardiovascular activities. Deliberately consuming a much higher ratio of carbohydrate to protein, however, can hinder performance, because your muscles don't get the protein they need to get and stay strong. So that marathoner eats more pasta with meat sauce, ultimately taking in more calories from protein and fat in addition to carbohydrate in order to support the energy output of the sport. A competitive powerlifter might find that protein intake closer to 1 gram per kilogram of body weight gives him more energy. This is a slight increase over the current guidelines of .8 gram per kilogram of body weight, but nowhere near the recommendations of other diets that promise huge weight gains. Active people need more calories overall, not specifically from one fuel source.

Let's look at the components of a healthy diet in general and how eating well can specifically contribute to the success of your early-morning workouts.

Carbohydrate

Carbohydrate is basically sugar, made up of carbon, hydrogen, and oxygen, and this is called a simple sugar. The number of simple sugars that are linked together determines whether it is a simple or more complex sugar. Starch and fiber are carbohydrates that are composed of many simple sugars linked together. One gram of carbohydrate contains four calories. Complex forms of carbohydrate can be found in foods that are still in their natural, unrefined state, while simple sugars are the result of processing the food in various ways. Carbohydrates are important for brain function and are your body's favored fuel to provide it with energy for functioning.

During the last few years, carbohydrate has been scrutinized from many different angles. Various popular diets such as the Atkins and South Beach programs have brought attention to carbohydrate like never before. The original theory behind the Atkins diet was that if you kept your carbohydrate intake extremely low, your body would become more efficient at burning fat for fuel and thus you would lose weight. The problem with diets of this type is that your body needs carbohydrate for everyday fuel, and your brain in particular needs it to function. Fat is not the body's first choice for energy. Also, you need a constant, low level of carbohydrate in order to be able to burn fat efficiently. The saying "fat burns in a carbohydrate flame" is a metaphor that makes sense physiologically. Another limitation of extreme low-carbohydrate diets is that without enough carbohydrate in your system, along with using fat your body will also try to use protein for energy. Protein is also not your body's first choice for basic fuel. The breakdown of protein for fuel is taxing on your kidneys and liver; it's not a process your body is designed to sustain over a long period of time.

The concept of "good carbohydrate" versus "bad carbohydrate" has become mainstream because of the diets just mentioned. Instead of using the terms "good" and "bad," it is more sensible and realistic to think of carbohydrates in terms of whether they are complex or simple. This determines how quickly they are broken down in your body, which is indicated by a food's score on the glycemic index.

To understand this better, let's use an apple as an example. The apple in its whole, natural state has a skin on it; as you digest the fruit, that skin needs to be broken down along with the apple's flesh. This slows down the rate at which your body can convert the apple's carbohydrate to the simple sugar glucose, so the whole apple is low on the glycemic index. If you peel the apple and make applesauce out of it, the removal of the skin means that some of the fiber is lost. The food is more processed (in this case it literally goes through the food processor!) and in a sense is partly predigested for you; your body will not have to work very hard to break down the carbohydrate into simple sugars. The applesauce is therefore higher on the glycemic index than the raw apple. Now, if instead of making applesauce you juice the apple and throw away the pulp, the end product is even more processed. So the apple juice is higher on the glycemic index than the applesauce or the raw apple.

Pure sugar, a simple carbohydrate, is assigned a glycemic index of 100, because your body does not need to break it down any further. When you consume it, it causes your blood sugar to increase quickly. This can lead to the unsettling up-and-down cycle of energy that you might notice when you eat a processed food that's high in simple sugar, like licorice or other candies that so many people keep on their desks. Your energy seems to zoom up for a little while and then it crashes, at which point you reach for some more sweets to bring it back up. Carbohydrate that is less refined (less processed) retains more of the natural fiber content, takes longer to break down, and so tends to be lower on the glycemic index. The general principle to keep in mind is that the less processed a food is, the lower it is on the glycemic index and the better it is for you. Good choices for carbohydrate are brown rice; breads and pastas made from whole grains; and fruits and vegetables. In the morning, you might sometimes be tempted to eat something high on the glycemic index in order to get a quick burst of energy for your workout instead of going back to sleep. Actually, this isn't a good idea; the reason why, and some healthier food choices to prepare you for your early-morning workouts, will be discussed later in this chapter.

Fiber is one form of carbohydrate. Obtainable from plant sources, it makes up much of the structure of leaves, stems, and roots, as well as the skin and flesh of fruit and the husks of grains. Plant foods that have not been processed a lot maintain their high fiber content. Unlike other nutrients, fiber is not digestible, which contributes to a slower rate of metabolism, as we saw with the apple example. It acts like a sort of broom in your intestines, helping to clean out your insides as it moves through your digestive system. Fiber retains a considerable amount of water throughout the digestive process and therefore makes you feel full longer. This is a good tip if you want to lose weight. Getting plenty of fiber (25–30 grams per day) can help you feel less hungry during the day and help keep your colon healthy too.

Fat

Fat, or lipid, is another of the macronutrients necessary for good health. You need fat to keep hair and skin healthy, provide insulin for your vital organs, and transport the fat soluble vitamins A, D, E, and K. Fat is an important type of fuel in your diet, even if you feel it's not a desirable thing to see on your body. Its 9 calories per gram are what make it a good source of energy. If you were stranded on a desert island, having fat to eat would ensure you could stay alive longer!

Like a carbohydrate molecule, a fat molecule is made up of carbon, hydrogen, and oxygen. Fat, however, has a higher ratio of hydrogen to oxygen than carbohydrate. This is where the terminology of "saturated" and "unsaturated" fats comes in. Saturated fat is "saturated" with hydrogen atoms—it contains as many as possible. Unsaturated fat, on the other hand, has less than the maximum number of hydrogen atoms. In general, you can think of saturated fat as fat that is solid at room temperature. Animal products contain saturated fat, as do coconut and palm oil. Saturated fat can raise the level of cholesterol (especially the harmful kind discussed farther on) in your blood, which increases your risk of atherosclerosis. Atherosclerosis is a condition in which cholesterol-rich deposits, or plaque, form on the inner lining of the arteries. This in turn can increase your blood pressure, meaning that your blood needs to be pushed through your arteries with more force than is optimal. Because of the health problems associated with eating saturated fat, it is widely recommended that the majority of your fat intake be unsaturated—for example, in the form of vegetable oils, extra-virgin olive oil, and nuts and legumes. The fat in certain kinds of fish has received positive attention recently. Omega-3 fatty acids found in fish such as sardines and salmon are thought to help prevent blood clots from forming on the artery walls. They also seem to be beneficial in regulating the rhythm of your heart. In addition, these essential fatty acids are currently considered important in reducing the level of inflammation within the body. Inflammation may contribute to fat being deposited in your arteries as well as the deterioration of the lining in and around your joints, potentially leading to conditions such as arthritis, for example.

Trans fat is an important health concern that has been getting quite a lot of attention in the last couple of years. Trans fat is basically unsaturated fat that has been altered to enhance the shelf life of the many products it's added to. The process of chemical alteration actually changes many of the molecules from unsaturated to saturated. Trans fat has all the potentially harmful effects of naturally saturated fat, and it may also contribute to lowering the good cholesterol, or HDL, that unsaturated fat helps raise. (HDL aids in the battle against heart disease by removing stickier LDL cholesterol from the walls of the arteries and bringing it to the liver for secretion.) Trans fat is listed as "partially hydrogenated oil" on food labels. Manufacturers will soon be required to list the amount of trans fat in their products, and many already do so. Try to avoid it as much as possible.

As stated earlier, you should try to get less than 10 percent of your daily calorie intake from saturated fat and less than 30 percent of your calories from any type of fat. Let's put the earlier example in terms of how many actual grams of fat you should be eating. If we assume you eat 2,000 calories per day to maintain your current body weight, then 30 percent would be 600 calories. You would want no more than 600 calories from fat of any kind, and no more than 200 calories from saturated fat. Each gram of fat has 9 calories, so you would limit your fat calories to about 66 grams total (600 calories divided by 9 calories per gram equals 66.6 grams), and only 23 grams of saturated fat (200 calories divided by 9 calories per gram equals 22.2 grams). When you consider how much fat is in many popular fried and fast foods (sometimes one meal has more fat than is recommended for the entire day!), it's no surprise that there are so many overweight and unhealthy people in our society.

Fat as a fuel source is not the same thing as fat stored around your midsection or hips. Think of your stored body fat as the calories you ate and didn't use. Protein and carbohydrate are also stored as body fat if you eat more than you need. There is a big misconception about this in the fitness industry. The "fat burning" program options on cardiovascular machines have encouraged people to exercise at relatively low intensity levels, not burning as many calories as they could have during their workout. Exercising at a low intensity does mean you will use relatively more fat than carbohydrate as fuel for your workout, but if the workout lasts the same amount of time, the overall calorie expenditure will be lower because the intensity, along with the duration, is what determines how many calories you burn. Many people forget that if you are going to work at a lower intensity with cardiovascular exercise to lose weight, then you need to work for a longer period of time to burn more calories in general. This mistake can sabotage your well-intentioned efforts to lose body fat. The bottom line if you want to lose weight is that you should work as hard as you can, for as long as you can. You basically need to burn more calories than you eat. Each pound of body fat contains 3,500 calories of food that you have not used, so you need to create a deficit by either burning more calories, eating less, or a combination of both.

Protein

Protein is the foundation of your muscles, bones, skin, and hair and is in virtually every body part and tissue. Amino acids are the building blocks of protein. Some proteins contain all the essential amino acids required by the body and are therefore called *complete proteins*. Sources of complete protein are mostly animal products such as eggs, milk, meat, fish, and poultry. Eggs are the perfect example of a complete protein; they provide the optimal mixture of essential amino acids. *Incomplete proteins* are lacking in one or more of the essential amino acids. If you don't eat a lot of animal products, you need to combine and vary your food choices to get complete protein. Beans and rice, for example, combine to form complete protein.

Nutrition guidelines suggest an average of .8 gram of protein per kilogram of body weight. As stated before, this amount should make up about 10 percent of your total daily calories. One kilogram equals 2.2 pounds. If you weigh 140 pounds (64 kilograms), for example, you would need about 51 grams of protein each day (64 × .8). There are 4 calories in each gram of protein, so 51 grams times 4 calories in each gram comes out to 204 calories from protein. You would need a total of about 2040 calories per day to maintain your current weight.

The average American consumes more than the recommended level of protein. That is why I do not support the notion that you need extra protein if you want to build more muscle. As important as protein is, it's important to realize that muscle is actually made up of at least 70 percent water. If you want to build more muscle, your main concern should really be to eat more quality calories in general. The stimulus of weight training, combined with proper nutrition and hydration and getting enough sleep, will allow your body to build muscle as well as possible. Consuming a high percentage of protein relative to your whole diet can lead to an imbalance in which the ratio of carbohydrate to protein is too low. This means that for energy your body has to rely on protein, which is not its preferred fuel source. Breaking down protein for energy is stressful to the liver and kidneys, as mentioned earlier, and it increases the nitrogen in your body above healthy levels.

You'll often see protein shakes and nutrition bars for sale at the gym and in health food stores. The nutrition bars that first came on the market were designed for endurance athletes and were composed mostly of carbohydrate, since this is the body's desired fuel source for activities lasting several hours. As excessive protein consumption became more popular, both to theoretically enhance muscle growth and to provide convenience food for people on the low-carbohydrate diets discussed earlier, different kinds of bars started being sold. These newer bars vary in their protein, carbohydrate, and fat content, but they were originally marketed to the bodybuilders who wanted a high proportion of calories from protein with as few calories as possible from carbohydrate. In the mid- to late 1990s, protein powders also came onto the market in full force. They are designed to be mixed with water, juice, or milk, and they come in numerous flavors and varieties. Concerning your morning strength workouts, you could argue that it might be helpful to have some kind of food bar available when you need something to eat in a hurry—if you wake up a little later than you wanted to, for example, or feel hungrier than normal. A good choice for a bar in this case would have a makeup of 60 percent carbohydrate, 30 percent fat, and 10 percent protein. I am not a food zealot, and I think the most important thing is balance—how you eat over the long run. It is certainly helpful sometimes to have something to grab and eat. But in general, I don't support eating food bars or drinking protein shakes. Remember that a piece of whole-grain bread with a teaspoon of peanut butter and one apple is a great choice, as is a slice of cheese with an apple. Even a couple of bites of leftover pizza can make a good substantial snack! Real food gives you natural vitamins and minerals, contains more fiber, and just tastes better than processed foods.

Water

More than half of your body weight is made up of water. Without taking in some form of water, you would die in a few days. It aids in digestion and food absorption and helps regulate body temperature. It helps carry nutrients and oxygen throughout the body, and helps your body get rid of toxins and waste.

In general, try to drink at least two quarts (slightly less than two liters) of water each day—this comes to about eight 8-ounce glasses. You also get water from food such as fruit and vegetables and drinks such as juices and tea. To avoid losing some of the water you consume because of caffeine's diuretic effect, try to stick mainly to caffeine-free herbal tea. If you don't get enough water during the day, you will get dehydrated, which can make you feel fatigued and irritable and even give you headaches. Being dehydrated also means that you'll have less energy in the morning to get up and work out.

If you find it difficult to drink enough water because you don't like the taste, try adding lemon or lime wedges to it. You might find that you prefer the taste of flavored water or seltzers to plain water. A great tip to stay aware of your water consumption is to get a bottle, determine how many times you have to fill it to reach a total of two quarts (again, this is equivalent to a bit less than two liters), and then wrap that many rubber bands around the bottom of the bottle. Each time you empty your bottle, you move one rubber band up to the top of the bottle. Then, when all the rubber bands are at the top, you know you've achieved your goal. The topic of water intake as it relates to your morning workouts is discussed later in this chapter.

Vitamins and Minerals

In contrast to the macronutrients discussed earlier, vitamins and minerals are called *micronutrients.* They are substances that we need in smaller amounts. Our bodies can't produce most of them, so we need to get these from the food we eat or from supplements. Vitamins are important in a number of biological processes. Among others, they aid in digestion, and they help your body absorb macronutrients and use them more efficiently. Minerals are important for healthy bones and teeth, and they help regulate the balance of fluids in your body. They are also important for the proper functioning of your nervous system. More and more, researchers are seeing vitamins and minerals as important in fighting cancers and other diseases such as arthritis.

According to organizations such as the National Institutes of Health, you can get all the vitamins and minerals you need from food. The challenge is to eat enough high-quality food to get these important nutrients. Processing food reduces its vitamin and mineral content. With the busy lifestyles that many of us lead, finding the time to buy and prepare food in a healthy manner can be very difficult. Try to get as many nutritious whole foods as possible in your diet. If you can't get all your nutrients from food, then consider taking a multivitamin to supplement your diet. If you are eating well and getting plenty of sleep but still feel fatigued in the morning when you get up to work out, it's possible that you are deficient in certain nutrients. In that case, or if you have any other special concerns, it's a good idea to consult a nutritionist.

Eating for a Better Morning Workout

Now that we've covered the basics of good nutrition and hydration and you know what to eat and drink for optimal results, let's explore the issue of what to eat and drink before, during, and after your workout.

Before Your Workout

The old saying that one should eat like a king in the morning, a prince in the middle of the day, and a pauper in the evening is a great way to think about your eating habits as they relate to your morning exercise. In fact, we should all eat this way, since from morning until late afternoon is when we are generally the most active and need the benefits of good nutrition. As your day draws toward its close, you don't need as many calories to function. Working out in the morning means you need even more energy at the beginning of the day so that you can get the most out of your routines and not feel tired because of poor nutrition.

Let's start with when you wake up. After you've been sleeping all night, your blood sugar levels are at their lowest point; your last meal was quite a few hours ago. Since your body and brain need a constant supply of carbohydrate, you are in a deficit as soon as you wake up. Because of this, it is important to eat something to get your blood sugar elevated and avoid feeling sluggish or light headed during your morning workout. Being told to eat before a morning workout can mean different things to different people. I once had a personal training client take my advice to eat some breakfast before our training session. He came in the next time after eating a huge bagel with a ton of cream cheese—it was no surprise that he was too full and felt uncomfortable during the workout. I guess I should have been clearer in my explanation! You want to eat something substantial, but fairly light.

If you have enough time in the morning, it would be great to eat something as much as one hour before your workout. That way your blood sugar can increase, your body can adapt to the food starting to be digested, and your energy level goes up without making you feel too full or too empty. This can be practical if you go to a gym to work out, since an hour might pass between the time you wake up and the time you get there. For many people, however, this advice can be impractical. If you work out at home, you might prefer to start exercising right away in the morning and not want to get up extra early just to eat something.

No matter where you do your morning workouts, do at least try to eat as soon as possible after waking up. A combination of carbohydrate, fat, and protein will give you the energy to get going. A piece of whole-grain bread with a little peanut butter on it is a good choice. That way you get your carbohydrate for energy, your fat to fill you up a little, and your protein. Some other good options are a small serving of whole-grain cereal with low-fat milk or even a small portion of your leftover dinner, such as stir-fried brown rice with seafood. How about a cup of low-fat yogurt with a banana? Or do you feel better if you eat a bowl of oatmeal before your morning workout? As suggested earlier, the best way to find out what works for you is to experiment and record your habits and how you feel. The one thing you definitely don't want to do in the morning is eat something very high in simple sugar or simple carbohydrate, like processed fruit juice or leftover white rice. This would make your blood sugar go up too quickly, giving you initial energy but soon leaving you feeling empty and sluggish—you don't want that in the middle of your walking lunges at 7 a.m.!

During Your Workout

You should have water with you during your workout. Your body needs to stay hydrated as you exercise, and this will save time looking for a water fountain if you are outdoors or at the gym. Drink several ounces (a big swallow equals approximately one ounce) every 15 to 20 minutes, and definitely anytime you are thirsty. Sport drinks have gotten very popular over the years because of creative marketing, but they are not necessary for a morning strength routine. What they offer is basically sugar and electrolytes designed to replenish minerals you lose through sweating, such as potassium. This is important for long cardiovascular workouts that last several hours, but not necessary for strength or even cardio workouts that last an hour or less. Using these drinks will only add extra calories to your diet, and because they are high in simple sugar to increase the rate of absorption, they contribute to the unnecessary cycle of your blood sugar peaking and crashing.

After Your Workout

After you've finished exercising, try to avoid rushing to work and then not eating for several hours. Since you work out in the morning, your daily food intake will not be made up of three traditional meals. The food you eat before and after your workout can be thought of as a two-part breakfast. It's important to eat after your strength workout, because you need to replenish the glycogen stores in your muscle cells and liver. Glycogen is stored sugar, which is what you used for energy during your workout, along with the small amount of food you ate to get going beforehand. Increasing the glycogen uptake into your muscles relatively quickly helps you recover faster and reap the gains you stimulated during your workout to build more muscle. Continue drinking water and ingesting fluids throughout the day.

During the rest of the day, your brain needs energy from the additional food you eat, and you are continuing to burn the calories you've already consumed. Eating a good lunch will help keep your blood sugar regulated and your energy up. Again, it's good to have a combination of protein, fat, and carbohydrate.

Salad with vegetables and grilled seafood is a great option. Half a sandwich on whole-grain bread with lean meat and mustard is also a good choice. Try to add a piece of fruit to your meal for extra nutrients. Getting calories from good, quality food consistently throughout your day will keep your body nourished so that you can recover from the morning workout and have enough stored energy to do the next one.

As a morning exerciser, you don't need many calories late in the day, so your dinner should be relatively light. Dinner is a good time to have something like fresh greens and lots of vegetables in a salad, with a piece of grilled chicken or other protein. Think about what you've eaten over the course of the day and determine whether anything important was missing. For example, if you went to a lunch party for a coworker where a pasta dish without much protein was served, then try to eat a bit more protein that night to make up for it, perhaps by making a scrambled egg white. If you skipped your veggies during the day, then have a few extra servings with your evening meal. The worst thing you can do in terms of being ready for your workout the next morning is to overeat late at night, right before you go to bed. This will disrupt your sleep and make you feel less motivated to get up the next day.

Life is not perfect, and sometimes we make poor food choices because of work or social situations. Other times we deliberately choose to have something like barbecue wings or a cheeseburger as a treat! Rather than beating yourself up because your diet isn't flawless, you need to balance things out so that when you look back at your eating habits over a week, you will see that overall you ate sensibly and kept to the diet recommended here. This, along with taking good care of yourself by getting enough sleep and paying attention to your other daily habits, will ensure the success of your morning routines.

Motivation to Keep Moving

This section covers some ways you might want to consider to keep your workouts fresh, fun, and always challenging. They will help you stay enthusiastic about getting up in the morning to work out for the long run. This section also includes a few tips in case you need a little kick in the gluteus maximus to stay on target! The importance of exercising through those times of life that are truly out of your control and very stressful is explored. Internalizing this knowledge and sticking with your program during such times is extremely beneficial for your well-being in general, as well as for your fitness level.

One way to keep your motivation up with your morning strength workouts is to change your routines. You can change the goal of the routine, the length of the workout, or both. For example, each time you work out, try a new 20-minute routine—first the one for strength, then the one for size, and so on until you finish them all. Then, if time permits, you can do all the 30-minute routines, and move on to the 45-minute routines. Cycling through the workouts in chapters 6 through 9 would constantly challenge your body in new ways as you alter the weight, the number of repetitions, and the equipment you use. This would ensure that you wouldn't get bored doing the same routine over and over. It would also mean that your body would always be adjusting to different movement patterns, which challenges your neuromuscular system and also decreases your chance of injury, since it prevents you from overtraining particular muscles or joints.

Another way to keep your routines interesting is to change the variables discussed in chapter 5. One variable you can change is the angles. That means when the exercise is a row with a cable, you can adjust the cable one morning so that you're pulling from above you; the next time you could adjust the cable so you are pulling from straight ahead; and the next time you could pull from below. This kind of variation will keep your workouts fresh and stimulate your mind.

Now and then, however, you may experience a lack of motivation some mornings, even if you have the best of intentions. Why does this happen? I guess the simplest answer is *life*—just the everyday stress of life! Perhaps you are feeling a little stressed because of something that happened the day before. Maybe you got a phone call the previous night and had to take care of something unexpectedly. Maybe you worked later than you anticipated, and after doing the necessary chores at home you didn't get to sleep as early as you meant to. If these things happen, here are some suggestions that might help.

If you are up late at night and know that you might need some extra motivation to get up the next morning with less than optimal sleep, you can put your alarm clock close enough to hear it, but far enough away so that you have to get up out of bed to turn it off. Once you are up, just keep moving until you are ready for your workout. Another great tip to get you moving more easily is to sleep with your workout clothes on. That way there's one less thing to do in the morning. Finally, when the alarm rings and you simply don't feel like getting up, try this. Be aware of the thoughts running through your head. Maybe you hear yourself complaining that you don't feel like doing this, but at the same time you hear another voice saying, "Get up and start getting ready!" I call this arguing with yourself and winning. Here's the thing: You know that as soon as you get going and start exercising you will be fine. You can also make a deal with yourself that if you don't feel like continuing your workout after the first 15 minutes, you can stop. In my 23 years of working with people, this has rarely happened.

If you like to have your coffee as you get ready to go to the gym, you can preset the machine if you have the kind that allows you to, or if not you can at least put the coffee and water in the night before to save time. There are other, more external motivational tools that might work for you as well. Perhaps one of your friends would like to work out with you in the morning. You don't even have to do the actual workout together—just agree to meet and go together to the gym, where each of you will do your own workout. When you make an agreement with someone, you feel accountable; you won't want to disappoint your friend by not showing up.

There are, of course, times in our lives when something extremely stressful happens, such as the death of a loved one, a career change, divorce, moving, and so on. These times can be challenging to us emotionally, mentally, and financially. Unfortunately, exercise routines are sometimes the first habit we drop when we're under severe stress. When you find yourself in a situation like this, think about all the benefits you appreciate from your morning workouts. It's sometimes even a good idea to write this down; it can help you relax and focus. Remember that you feel better about yourself when you do your morning routines regularly. Remind yourself of the terrific goals you have met, or maybe some weight that you've lost because you committed to your morning routines. Exercise releases endorphins, natural opiates that contribute to a general sense of well-being. Try to really focus on the positive aspects of your morning program, and make a commitment to yourself again.

Remember also that taking time for your exercise program means you will be better able to take care of anyone else who is depending on you right now. Working out first thing in the morning is vital, since you may have to take care of unexpected things during the day and will be unable to exercise later. Keep in mind that the workouts in this book give you the flexibility to shorten your workout if committing to less time is an option you feel comfortable with. Working out in the morning contributes positively to your mind-set as well as your health—it really helps you deal both physically and emotionally with the stress of whatever is going on right now. Remember to take time to take care of yourself!

2

Your Workout Environment

‖‖

Working out in the morning requires you to be a little more organized and prepared than working out later in the day. It can be hard enough sometimes just to make time to eat breakfast, get to work on time, and do everything else you need to do at the beginning of the day! Investing a little time and energy into making your workout space efficient can help you fit your exercise program into your lifestyle. This chapter will show you how to do that.

Your workout space can take many different forms. You might exercise in a traditional multipurpose health club that has more than one floor and more than one place where you can get your strength workout done. Perhaps you go to this gym regularly for cardio workouts or classes as well as your strength workouts. Or maybe you exercise at a small gym, where you need to be more aware of others around you, and someone else might be using the equipment you want. The workouts in this book can be adapted so that you can use whatever equipment is available; this is discussed further on. Perhaps you don't want or aren't able to join a gym at this point and instead work out at home, or even outside when weather permits. This chapter will discuss the pros and cons of different workout spaces and give you tips for getting a great workout, no matter where you are.

Strength Training at Home

Every workout location has its advantages and disadvantages, and it's important to weigh these in deciding where to do your morning strength routines. A major advantage of working out at home is that it is convenient. Time is precious in the morning, and not having to go to the gym and back will give you more of it to spend on your workouts. If you always go to a gym to work out, time constraints might mean that you can't try any of the 60-minute routines in this book; this is less of a concern if you work out at home. It's also a good idea to have a workout that you can do at home in case you wake up too late to make it to the gym or your plans change for some other reason—that way you won't have to skip your workout for the day. Having a workout space at home is also convenient on the weekend. It means you don't need to take so much time away from your family, and it helps you stay consistent with your fitness program.

Working out at home can also contribute to your self-esteem and self-image. Of course, making a commitment to exercise in the morning is an accomplishment in and of itself. Working out at home gives you extra reason to feel good about yourself, since it is arguably more difficult to feel motivated at home than when you have the external stimulus of the gym.

These advantages are balanced by the potential difficulties of exercising at home. Unless you have the space and money to buy several different types of equipment, you probably won't be able to vary your workouts at home as much as you could at a gym. The importance of varying your workout is discussed in chapter 5, but briefly, changing your routine keeps your body from getting too familiar with one movement or exercise. Challenging your joints and muscles in new ways by changing angles, using different equipment, and so on targets more muscle fibers and gets your joints used to being stressed in different positions. This enhances your ability to lift weight, helping you reach your strength goals more quickly. Lacking a variety of equipment at home could limit your workouts somewhat.

Another potential challenge of working out at home is that you might disturb people who live with you or around you. You need to be aware of others in your home who could find your workouts disruptive in the nice, quiet morning hours. If you have enough room, try to set up your workout space far away from anyone who is usually sleeping at that time of day. You should also consider whether your workouts could bother people who live above or below you—people who might hear your dumbbells banging on the floor over and over again! You should always set dumbbells down quietly, but just in case you forget once in a while, you need a rack or a thick mat or carpet on the floor where you can put the weights between sets without making too much noise.

Distraction can also be a problem when you work out at home. You are obviously motivated since you've made a commitment to exercise in the morning, but at home there are many things around you that could divert your attention. Potential distractions are very individual to you. Maybe you suddenly notice dirt on the floor of your home and start cleaning that up instead of continuing with your workout. Others might tend to get sidetracked by the telephone, the computer, other people, or any number of things. It's smart to prepare for these distractions ahead of time so you can deal with them successfully—or avoid them altogether. If the phone rings during your workout, for example, can you let it ring, or do you feel compelled to answer it? If you answer it, do you feel comfortable telling the caller that you can't talk at the moment, or are you tempted to get into a conversation? Maybe you should just turn the phone off during your workouts.

If you live with other people, they can prove to be either a distraction or a source of support for your exercise program. You could enlist their help in leaving you the time to get your workout done and even develop some kind of reward for your kids if they don't disturb you. On the other hand, if time permits, you can invite your kids to work out with you. Ask them to try some of the core exercises that are done with just body weight. One of my clients told me that I helped her son learn to count by asking him to count along with us as she did her exercises in the living room. Working out in front of and with your kids is a great way to instill in them the habit of exercise—as well as the feeling that it's not an unusual occurrence!

Working out at home takes some planning—it's not as easy as just walking into a gym, buying a membership, and heading for the machines. There are several considerations to keep in mind. The physical space you exercise in can be a big factor in how comfortable you feel during your workout and how motivated you feel when you get up in the morning. It's worth putting a little time into arranging your home workout space. Seeing your weight bench covered with unfolded clean laundry might not be the most inspiring way to get going in the morning. If you organize an area of your home either as a permanent space for working or at least as a spot where your equipment is easily accessible, you'll be able to get to your routine with less wasted time. Here are some suggestions for optimizing your workout at home.

Space to Move

If you can set aside a workout space of about 10 feet by 10 feet (about 3 by 3 meters), you have enough space for a bench, a stability ball, a few pieces of tubing (also known as bands), some dumbbells, and room for you to move a little. If you have the extra space, keep this area designated for your workouts only, which will also motivate you since you'll see it all the time. If you don't have enough space to devote this area solely to your morning routines, then you need to have some storage space where you can keep your equipment in between the days you use it. This can turn into a hassle—you might find yourself having to dig deep into the closet to find those dumbbells. Planning ahead to avoid this scenario is key. Put the items out the night before so they will be ready for you in the morning. If you have the space, you can buy a rack for your dumbbells; if you don't, you need to have a mat or a carpet that you can put on the floor during your workout, as explained previously. You also need either a mat, a rug, or even a thick towel for the floor exercises. Just be careful if using a towel when you do standing exercises as it could be slippery.

Clear away any objects that might cause you to trip or twist an ankle, such as toys, shoes, and the like. Also clear away any clutter that might encourage you to lose your focus. Have a towel handy, and fill up your water bottle in advance. On a safety note, if you live alone, make sure you have a plan in case you need emergency help. Either make sure that your neighbors are around when you work out and could hear you calling out, or have a phone close by to use just in case you feel ill or drop a weight on your foot!

Lighting

Think of the days when you wake up in the morning to find the sun shining brightly into your bedroom. You feel more energized on those days than when you wake up and the weather is dark and dreary, don't you? Light in the morning, either natural sunlight or artificial light that simulates it as closely as possible, helps you reset your body's natural clock so that you can focus on your morning workout instead of trying to wake up. If you have a window in your workout space, try to have drapes or a shade that you can open in the morning; if you prefer to keep the window covered, you can get a thin, light-colored curtain that will still let in some natural light. If there's no window or if it's dark out when you get up (as can often be the case in wintertime), make sure you have a good light so that the room is pretty bright. If you don't, you might want to buy another lamp. You can even buy full-spectrum lightbulbs that mimic sunlight.

Ventilation

It's more pleasant to exercise in the morning if you're not doing it in a space with stale air, so make sure you have proper ventilation in your workout area. Think of the times when you open the windows, fresh air streams into the room, and you take a deep breath. You feel great, right? Compare this sensation with the way you feel in a room with no windows or with air that feels like the windows haven't been opened for a long time. The first scenario is much more conducive to waking up. Having fresh air circulating through the area where you exercise means you'll get plenty of oxygen into your lungs and on its way to your muscles, helping you feel alert and ready to work. Try to set up your workout space in an area that has cross-ventilation, with air that moves from one window or door to another. If this is not an option, then get a fan to increase circulation.

Temperature

The ideal temperature for working out is approximately 68 to 72 degrees Fahrenheit (20–22 degrees Celsius). It will be easier to get started with your workout in the morning if the room is the right temperature, neither too warm nor too cold. A room that is too warm can make you feel lethargic, especially if your bed is close in sight! If it's too cold, on the other hand, you won't warm up efficiently and will risk injury. Warming up is discussed in detail in chapter 4, but basically, if don't get your blood going through your body to warm up your joints and muscles, you're more likely to pull a muscle. A warm-up is necessary to get your blood sugar circulating and to get your joints lubricated and ready to handle the weight you are going to lift. Exercising is all about muscles contracting, or shortening, and then relaxing, or lengthening, over and over again. If the muscle fibers and joints are not warmed up, the muscle fibers don't shorten and lengthen efficiently, making it easier to overstretch or pull a muscle. This is particularly important since you are exercising in the morning. If you exercise later in the day when you've been up and about for a while, the temperature in the room is not so crucial, since you're already warm from the inside out. Try to make sure the room is heated properly, but if you still feel a little cool as you start your warm-up, it's a good idea to layer a light shirt on top of what you usually wear and take it off as you get going with your workout.

Music or Other Sounds

This is a very personal choice. What motivates you while you are working out? Does a quiet environment allow you to focus better on what you are doing, or does it make it harder to wake up and get going? Perhaps you like to listen to a radio station with some balance between news and music. You can also record a special CD or tape that is perfectly timed for your favorite workout, 30, 45, or however many minutes long, consisting of whatever music gets you moving. You can put the songs in the exact order you like. For example, if you want a little more inspiration at the beginning of your routine, then put that music first. Or you might be someone who likes the music to really match the workout. In that case, choose some quieter music for the warm-up and beginning of your routine, with the more energetic songs from the middle to the end. Finding the right music or other audible stimulus can help you have fun and get the most out of your morning routines.

Equipment

You can do many of the workouts in this book with one bench, a few sets of dumbbells, some pieces of tubing, a medicine ball, and a stability ball. You can also substitute other items for equipment you don't have. If you lack the space for the foam roller discussed in chapter 4, you can put three tennis balls in a sock and use that for the self-myofascial release instead. If you don't have a medicine ball, you can use a dumbbell in its place. If you don't have a stationary bicycle, you can get some cardiovascular intervals by using a jump rope.

Your dumbbells should vary from being light enough for overhead presses to heavy enough for a set of lunges or step-ups. There are also adjustable dumbbells on the market that attach to a device that lets you "click in" the weight you want so that more or less weight comes with each dumbbell as you lift it up.

The tubing should be strong enough to provide resistance for upper-body exercises such as rows. There should be something stable in the room, such as a column or a doorknob, that you can either attach the tubing to or wrap the tubing around. You should be able to lengthen the tubing to 1.5 times its resting length; if that doesn't give you enough resistance, you should get a thicker piece of tubing.

If you can get a stability ball, you will find it a wonderful tool for challenging your balance and core integrity. A stability ball should be big enough that your knees are at right angles when you sit on it. Keep it fully inflated. You can buy a stability ball that comes with a pump, or you can just use a bicycle pump if you have one.

If you have the space and the money, you might consider buying a cable column for your workout area at home. Many manufacturers produce these, and they are great for doing the upper-body exercises in this book. They often are designed with a bar across the top that you can use for chin-ups and hanging leg raises. You can also check to see if you can buy used exercise equipment somewhere nearby. Frequently gyms are looking for someone to buy machines they no longer want even though they are still in good condition. Health clubs are always trying to stock up on the latest things, and this might be a way for you to get a sturdy piece of equipment without spending much money. There are also companies that specialize in refurbishing used equipment and reselling it.

Another type of purchase to consider if you have the space and the money is a cardio machine such as a stationary bike, an elliptical machine, or a treadmill to complement your morning strength routines. There are many companies that make cardio machines for home use. These are designed to take up less space than the machines you'll find in health clubs, but the biggest difference is the degree of sturdiness. Machines built for commercial use have to be very strong to withstand the hours of use (and abuse) they will likely receive. This is why when you shop for home machines, they might look a little wimpy in comparison. Just be sure to do your research on the warranty that comes with a machine. If it covers both parts and maintenance for several years, you can feel assured that the manufacturer is not planning for the machine to break down in response to consistent home use. Make sure you always turn off the cardio equipment after you use it, and you should also unplug it if there are others in your home who might wander onto it and start it by accident.

If you only work out at home and don't have a multistation gym machine, you'll have to make slight changes to some of the routines. For example, if the exercise is a leg press, choose another leg exercise that you can do at home, such as a step-up or one of the many lunges or squats. If the exercise is a row done on a machine, then do the row standing with the tubing instead, or the single-arm row with a dumbbell and your bench. You can buy bars that fit tightly inside a doorway and stay in place by friction, with no need for bolts or screws. This is an easy way to be able to do exercises like chin-ups and hanging leg raises at home.

Outdoor Strength Workouts

Exercising outdoors is quite a different experience from working out at home or in a gym. It brings you back to when you were a kid happily playing outside. Our lifestyles are so sedentary that we have become removed from the natural feeling of movement and exercise. We're so used to the idea of exercising in a certain building called a health club that we forget how many places there are to exercise! I think of this when I see parents or caregivers sitting on benches in a playground while the children are playing. Why can't the grown-ups play (or work out) too? Moving your workout outside gives you the opportunity to do this. Outdoor workouts are also excellent if you travel a lot and like to run for your cardio exercise. You can go for a run, and if you find a spot to do the exercises listed later in this section, you will have a great routine.

If you choose to work out outdoors, it's best to do it when it is light out, both for reasons of safety and so that you can see what you're doing. Being outdoors during the day will expose you to natural sunlight, which is important in regulating your natural body clock. This will help you sleep better at night and wake up more easily for your next workout. Being outside will also enable you to get lots of energizing fresh air.

When preparing for your workout outside, have necessary items ready to go, such as your car keys, ID, cell phone, emergency information, and audio equipment, if you like to listen to music during your workout. Remember to take your water bottle with you, and perhaps a snack you can eat on the way out or back. Some good choices for snacks are nuts and fruit, low-fat cheese, or half a sandwich. (This is also discussed in chapter 1.) Take any equipment you need, such as tubing or a medicine ball. Be sure to wear shoes with good support for the jumping exercises.

I like to call outdoor workouts "playground routines," since they are easily done in a playground where there are a climbing apparatus and objects of different heights. If you don't have such a place near your home, try to find an area with a bench, stairs, or a wall about knee height. Here are some examples of how you can use the props in a playground or other outdoor area to do the exercises described in this book:

- Climbing apparatus: You can use this to do chin-ups or hanging leg raises.
- Bench: You can use this to do regular, walking, and plyometric push-ups, as well as step-ups.
- Post or other stable object: You can use this to wrap a piece of tubing around for pulling and pushing exercises.

The following outdoor workout is a challenging routine that balances the goals of muscular strength and size, since you are using your body weight against gravity for several of the exercises. The sequence takes about 20 minutes to complete. After you do one set of each exercise, repeat the entire sequence once or twice, depending on how much time you have. Rest in between exercises to catch your breath.

- Movement prep warm-up. Page 55.
- Hanging leg raise: Page 178. Work up to 15 reps.
- Squat jump: Page 198. Work up to 10 reps.
- Regular or negative chin-up: Page 145. Work up to 10 reps.
- Plyometric push-up against horizontal bar on climbing apparatus or wall: Page 150. Work up to 10 reps.
- Jump lunge: Page 205. Work up to 10 reps.
- Row with tubing coming from in front: Page 137. Work up to 25 reps.
- Chest press with tubing coming from behind: Page 154. Work up to 25 reps.

Pay attention to the weather report and prepare accordingly the night before. An outdoor strength workout requires more layered clothing than an outdoor cardio workout. Cardiovascular exercise generally warms your body up more rapidly than strength training, because it has you moving more limbs at the same time and in a continuous manner. You probably have noticed this when you go for a run. In strength workouts, you are not rhythmically moving your whole body at the same time. Don't worry—you will get nice and warm, but it won't happen as quickly. So if it's cool outside, be sure to layer your clothing for your morning workout. You'll be doing your strength workout at a specific place, so you can just put your jacket down after you warm up. The layer closest to your body should absorb perspiration and keep the sweat away from your skin. Many brands of workout clothes use fabrics designed to do this. The outer layer should keep out the cold and moisture.

Outdoor strength workouts can be tough and even unsafe when the weather is cold or otherwise inclement. You can slip if there is ice, mud, or snow on the ground, and thick gloves are cumbersome at best when you are trying to do pull-ups or hold on to a medicine ball. If you know the weather will be bad, it's best to plan to use one of the other workouts in this book. Outdoor programs in the warmer months take some preparation too. Make sure you have a layer to take off as you warm up. You will also need extra water when exercising outdoors in the warmer weather. Being thirsty is a definite sign that you need more water; in fact, you should try to stay hydrated enough not to reach the point of thirst. If you often exercise outdoors in warm weather, you should weigh yourself before and after a workout. If you've lost weight, that is an indication that you didn't drink enough water before, during, and after your workout. This is especially important in the morning, since you have been sleeping all night and might not have enough fluid inside you. You should avoid exercising in hot weather unless you are conditioned to it.

Strength Training in the Gym

If you are the kind of person who feels more motivated exercising away from home, the gym is a great destination for your morning workouts. Sometimes it's helpful to have a special place to inspire you to devote time and energy to exercising. Belonging to a gym is a signal to yourself that your fitness program is important. It can also encourage you to get the most out of each workout, since once you've taken the time to get there you might as well do the entire routine instead of stopping in the middle of your core exercises! If your health club is along the route of your morning commute, stopping there on the way to work can save you time in the morning. This is a good option if you are fairly well organized—you will have to get your work clothes and everything else you need for the rest of the day prepared ahead of time. Another big advantage of going to the gym is that it means you will usually have access to all the equipment you need for your workout.

If you go to a gym for your strength workout, there are a few things to keep in mind. It's useful to have a place in your home where you can put everything you'll need to take with you in the morning. Have your transportation items ready to go—car keys, bike lock keys, bus or train card, and so on. Have your music equipment ready, with the battery charged. Fill your water bottle and either keep it with everything else or put it in the refrigerator to get cold. If you refrigerate it, you might want to keep a reminder by your other items so you don't forget it in the morning. If you decide to take a bar or banana with you, keep that with the other items as well (the issue of eating before and after your workouts is discussed in chapter 1).

Have your workout clothes ready to go before you go to bed the night before. You might even find it helpful to sleep in some of your workout clothes! Keep your sneakers with the other items to take with you. If you know you are going to do some jumping or plyometric exercises in your workout, make sure that your sneakers are not old and worn out. If you can rent a locker at your gym, it can help you stay organized. You could keep a pair of sneakers in the locker, along with shower supplies and maybe an extra pair of underwear.

When you go to the gym to exercise, think ahead about where you are going to do your workout. Know where the different kinds of equipment are set up and plan accordingly. Do you need the free weights today, or the machines? Maybe your routine will use the stability ball and cables. Some places duplicate their equipment, which lets you avoid crowded areas. Your health club might have one spot devoted just to free weights and a few more free weights located right next to the machines. So, if you know you are going to use mostly free weights today, go to the area set apart for them instead of to the place by the machines—that way there's a better chance that the dumbbells you need will be available. Thinking ahead like this can save you a lot of time.

You also need to consider how to keep track of the exercises in your routine. You can either take this book with you, photocopy the workout you have chosen for the day, or just write it down on a piece of paper. Remember that you can always make changes to your workout if you want to. This is discussed in detail in chapter 5. It does help, though, to have a general plan in mind so that when you get to the gym you are less likely to be distracted or waste time.

Exercising in the morning is all about efficiency. A potential distraction at the gym is running into others you might want to chat with. If you are the kind of person who is easily tempted to talk to others instead of working out, avoid crowded areas where you are likely to see people you recognize. If you do see someone you know, just say hello and motion or say that you need to keep moving to finish your workout in a timely manner. Wearing headphones (whether or not you are actually listening to music) is a great way to let others know that you probably do not want to talk right now.

Some additional options at the gym are strength training classes and private or small group personal training. Classes can offer a number of benefits. They are usually designed to progress logically from start to finish, so you get your warm-up, strength training component, and stretching at the end. If you're the kind of person who is liable to end a workout early because you feel bored or tired, doing a class once in a while is great to keep on pace. One potential drawback to group strength classes is that they often don't use enough weight to be challenging unless you do lots of repetitions. This is fine, however, if your main goal is endurance, or just for variety once in a while.

As a professional personal trainer, I believe that personal training is a valuable service. I base my philosophy on the idea that the client should be an active participant in the process, and that is exactly what this book helps you do. You can hire a personal trainer when you begin your new program to help you tweak it for your individual needs, or you can consult someone once in a while to help you stay on track.

The information in this chapter should allow you to make an educated choice about where to work out in the morning, how to stay organized and efficient, and how to be inspired by your environment. Evaluate your needs and preferences carefully, and you will discover what works best for you.

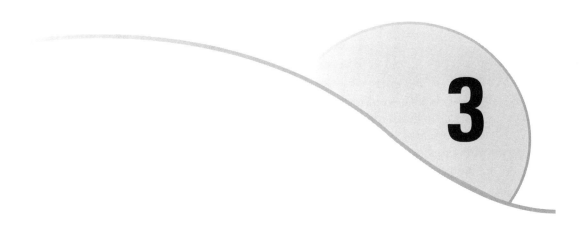

Selecting Your Equipment

The great variety of equipment that is available for strength training these days gives us unprecedented options to meet our goals and plenty of ways to vary our programs. Choosing among all the different alternatives, however, can be a confusing and sometimes even overwhelming process.

People often ask me which machines or pieces of equipment will work them hardest and give them the best results. In terms of strength training, the main point to remember is that the only thing your body knows is resistance. When you put resistance against a movement powered by your muscles, you stimulate those muscles to become stronger, bigger, and able to work over a longer period of time. This is the simple principle of strength training; what complicates matters is that there are many different ways to get resistance. Once you understand the advantages and disadvantages of some of the various ways to work against resistance, you will be better able to pick the workouts offered in chapters 6 through 9 to suit your preferences and goals. You will also be able to make changes to these workouts if you don't have (or don't like) the equipment suggested in a specific routine.

Body Weight

The most fundamental form of resistance we as human beings encounter is gravity. Gravity is always pulling us toward the earth. Simply pulling or pushing our bodies away from gravity is an exercise! This can be a big advantage for working out in the morning, especially when you are working at home or outdoors instead of going to the gym. The power workouts in this book that incorporate body-weight exercises are great routines that you can do anywhere.

To understand the advantages of body-weight exercises that work against gravity, let's use the push-up as an example. When you lie facedown and push away from the floor, you are pushing against the force of gravity, which wants to keep you on the floor. The muscles that push you away—your pectoralis major, or pecs; anterior deltoids; and triceps—have to contract in order to do this, and they get a good workout in the process.

Besides stimulating our muscles, working against gravity creates impact when we step onto the ground and then away again. This action is very important for bone and joint integrity. Bones are constantly regenerating, and the force of impact helps stimulate this process. A good way to think about working against gravity is to picture a simple movement such as walking up a flight of stairs. Each time you lift up your right leg to get to the next step, you are moving against gravity. Then, as you place your right foot on the step, you need to push down into the ground in order to propel your body in the opposite direction so that your left foot comes up off the step, ready to move on. When you work against gravity in a similar exercise such as walking lunges, all the parts of your body from the floor up need to work together. For some people this is a simple maneuver, but for deconditioned folks, walking up a long flight of stairs isn't much fun!

Using your body weight against gravity gives you an indication of what your relative strength is. *Relative strength* means your strength relative to your body weight. If you were only able to do exercises in which you had to lift or move your body against gravity, you would get stronger relative to how much you weigh. This is why boot-camp workouts have been so popular through the years—they make you move your own body, which for many people is quite difficult. Compare this with a typical bodybuilding routine. The bodybuilder's goal is to develop muscular size, strength, and symmetry, without regard to using that size and strength in any particular movement.

Your body is put together like a chain, with each muscle and the fibers that wrap around it connecting to the next muscle across the same or the next joint. So in a body-weight exercise like a lunge, where you step forward on the floor, your sensory organs in your joints and muscle fibers sense where you are and what you need to do to either gain or keep your balance. Your nervous system then automatically tells your muscles where you are in space, causing your foot and ankle to make any adjustments to stabilize your body to keep you balanced and to get ready for the next step. This kind of practice gives your body an opportunity to become more efficient at working as a whole in everyday life (so important in these days of sitting too much at work and in the car!) and trains it to react appropriately in different situations, like stepping off a curb the wrong way or having to pick something up while turning around to answer someone. The morning workouts that incorporate body-weight exercises in chapters 6 to 9 will get your body moving in this way.

Free Weights

Free weights (dumbbells and barbells) add resistance to exercises, thus stimulating your muscles to gain in strength, size, or endurance, depending on how you tailor the exercises to your individual goals. Gravity is still pulling straight down, so sometimes when using free weights you have to manipulate your body's position relative to gravity in order to get a good exercise.

Let's look at a chest-press exercise, which is essentially the same pushing exercise as a push-up, working your pecs, anterior deltoids, and triceps. If you stand with a dumbbell in each hand and hold your arms up and out in order to perform the exercise, you will not be targeting the muscles you want as effectively as if you lie down on your back (supine) and push the dumbbells up away from gravity. Since gravity is pulling straight down, the muscles that are lined up against that force will be most challenged. In the standing example, your shoulder muscles, or deltoids, would do the most work just in order to hold the weights up.

Free weights are great tools to incorporate into a workout, because you can use them anywhere. Sometimes, though, a limiting factor comes into play: one's ability to hold the weights. When doing lunges, for example, it is difficult for some people to hold a dumbbell that's heavy enough to meet the needs of the exercise—for example, to reach fatigue in 8 to 10 repetitions. If you have trouble holding on to heavy weights, you might need to do more sets with a lighter weight, do another exercise first to fatigue the targeted body part, or do the exercise slower to get more time under tension.

So, which are better: body-weight exercises against gravity or free-weight exercises? The best answer is always "it depends." Neither is better; they are just different. Let's look at the push-up and chest press with dumbbells again. For many people, the chest press is harder. For starters, you need to be able to hold a dumbbell in each hand and negotiate the movement above your body. This is challenging until you learn the specific pattern you need to do the exercise. If you are limited in your wrist, elbow, or total-arm strength, then the weight you pick needs to be light enough for these areas to hold and might not be enough to overload your chest muscles. A push-up, on the other hand, is easier in terms of your wrist, elbow, and total-arm strength because you are pushing against the floor, which gives you more stability. The challenge with a push-up is the core strength in addition to the upper-body strength that you need to push your body away from gravity. You can make this easier by doing the push-up on your knees instead of toes, essentially making your body shorter.

If your goal is to increase pure strength with a weight you can lift, as well as to improve proprioception and your body's ability to work together as a whole, free weights are the way to go. Conversely, if your goal is to increase your relative strength, then picking a body-weight exercise instead of a free-weight exercise is a good choice. If you want to vary your program, then alternating the exercises is a great idea.

Machines

If your goal is to get your muscles bigger and stronger, and you're less concerned about your relative strength and how your whole body works together, then machines are a great choice. When you sit at a machine, you do not have to hold yourself up so much. The machine helps support your body, making it easier to lift heavier weights. If you like to work with machines and they will help you reach your goals, you can exchange the different exercises in this book, substituting machine exercises for body-weight or free-weight exercises.

When strength training on machines, you don't have to worry about your body position relative to gravity the way you do with body-weight or free-weight exercises. This is because the machine is an intricate, carefully designed system of cables, cams, and pulleys that allows you to lift plates off a weight stack to challenge your muscles. There are ways to adjust a machine's seat or movement arms to target more efficiently the muscles you are trying to work while supporting your body in the correct position.

To determine whether the seat and arm adjustments are correct for you, do the movement with your limbs first without using the movement arms of the machine. Then try to match it on the machine, adjusting the machine's parts until you can get the movement right. For example, when you use the seated-row machine, you begin the movement with your arms out in front of you a little below chest height, and then you pull your arms back, bending at your elbows. You pull back until your elbows are just past your body, forming about a 90-degree angle in their final position. To get an idea of the correct form, perform this movement without using the machine. Then, when you hold the grips of the machine (this exercise uses the vertical grips) and do the movement again, your arms should look and feel like they are doing the same movement. If your elbows get to 90 degrees before you pull them back very far, then the seat is too high. If when you pull back you can't even get to 90 degrees and you feel like you want to lift your arms up instead of moving them straight back, then the seat is too low.

If you are not familiar with a machine, take a few moments to determine where the settings for the seat and any other adjustments are. Be careful getting in and out of machines; also take note of any potential "pinch points" for your fingers—e.g., knobs that you have to pull or turn—and be careful when using them. When using machines, always remember to sit up tall and maintain good posture, keeping your core strong, your shoulders down and back without straining, and your head and neck neutral and not forward.

Cables

When you work with cables, the resistance comes from a weight stack, just as it does with a machine. The difference between cables and machines is that you can do a lot of exercises standing when you use cables, whereas most machine exercises involve sitting. Cables are beneficial for morning workouts if you are tired or just need to do a shorter routine, because using them works more of your body in one exercise. Also, standing exercises make you use your core more than you do when sitting on a machine, so cable exercises are a great choice if you want to focus on that during a particular workout, or just as a variation to include in your program now and then.

Cables that are not fixed at one spot are the best, because they let you adjust the height from which you work and thus the angle from which you pull. The cable exercises in this book ask you to pull from straight ahead, up above, or down below. A good integrated program constantly changes variables to keep your body working its muscles along different lines, never stagnating because of overly repetitive exercises. Making simple changes such as pulling from different angles will elicit a good response from your body and will make your routine more effective. This is great for early-morning workouts.

As with free weights, when you use cables you need to get your body in position to get the proper amount of resistance and create an angle that will target the right muscles. For example, when doing straight-arm pull-downs with a cable, you need to lean forward slightly from your hips to start the exercise with your uplifted arms forming a straight line with your torso, instead of standing straight up with your arms out of line with your body and raised only partway. Bending forward this way allows you to get full range of motion during the exercise.

Tubing

Tubing, along with medicine and stability balls (discussed next), is sometimes called a toy, because it can add an element of fun to your workout. Some of these tools originally came to the fitness arena via physical therapy, but by now they're pretty standard components of the equipment that health clubs buy. The terms *tubing* and *band* are sometimes used interchangeably, although I will differentiate between the two for the workouts in this book. The only exercise in this book done with a band is band walking, for the outer-hip muscles, described in chapter 12.

Tubing is a piece of stretchable plastic with one handle at each end. Tubes come in different colors; each color indicates a certain thickness and therefore a certain resistance. Since there is no consistency between manufacturers in their color coding, you need to feel each tube for yourself.

The resistance of the tubing comes into play when you lengthen it as you do the exercise. Begin the exercise at the point where you feel tension in the tubing before you begin the first repetition. The resistance will increase as you go through the desired range of motion, since the tubing is being stretched or lengthened. You can ultimately lengthen tubing to about 1.5 times its resting length. If you find you need to lengthen it more than that to get enough resistance for your desired set, choose a thicker piece of tubing that you'll have to work harder to stretch.

For safety's sake, do not just release the handles when you're done with the exercise. Let them go slowly so they don't snap back at you or at someone walking by. Also, before you use tubing, make sure that it doesn't seem dry or stiff; this could mean it has been kept outside too long and might break as you use it.

Having a couple of different pieces of tubing available is helpful in the morning routines. You can attach a piece of tubing to a machine in the gym and use it to do a set of horizontal rows for your posterior (rear) deltoids if the machine is being used. If you use tubing, you can adjust the angle from which you pull, which makes tubing a good alternative if the cables you need to use for an exercise are not adjustable.

Tubing is great for outdoor workouts, since it doesn't weigh much and you can do many different exercises with it. As we saw in the discussion of working out with free weights, it can sometimes be tricky to align the targeted muscles correctly against gravity. Tubing is a perfect way to avoid this problem, since you don't need to work against gravity when you use it. You can simply attach it to or loop it around a fixed object and pull!

Medicine Balls

Medicine balls have traditionally been used for sport-specific training, although they are a great addition to an integrated strength training program for several reasons. Just holding a medicine ball makes your hand, wrist, and entire arm work harder than when pulling on a grip on a machine, for example. This is terrific if you have relatively weak wrists and want to develop more integrity throughout the entire chain of your arm, as well as more upper-body strength in general. One of the limitations of our current lifestyle is that we simply don't have to use our upper bodies very much. We do too much sitting; we don't have to lift many things in our everyday lives beyond grocery bags and household items. There are different types of medicine balls, or med balls. Some bounce, and others do not. Some are easier to hold onto than others because of the outside material. Some have handles on them, enabling you to use them as dumbbells as well. For the workouts in this book, one or two medicine balls made from any material will work just fine. Pick one that is about 5 percent of your body weight and maybe another that is a little heavier than that.

The full-body warm-up in chapter 4 is a good way to use the medicine ball in your morning routines. By making you move your whole body together, it improves your coordination, and for the same reason it helps you feel wide awake more quickly and gives you energy as you go through the rest of your day.

Medicine balls are great for working on power, using exercises like throwing or pretending to throw the ball in different directions. This kind of exercise requires you to generate a lot of force in a short period of time and with a small range of motion—advantageous in the morning, since it means you're getting more work done in less time. If you are doing a power move like a throw or a pretend throwing movement, use a medicine ball that is 5 to 10 percent of your body weight. If the ball is too heavy, you'll find it hard to move the ball through space with enough energy to get the exercise stimulus you want. When in doubt, start with a lighter ball, since it's easy to pick a heavier one the next time.

Another way medicine balls can be useful is to provide resistance when you don't have a dumbbell—in a seated rotation exercise, for example. When you use a ball for this purpose, you should generally choose a heavier one than you would for power exercises.

Stability Balls

These large plastic balls look like they could be used on the beach for a game of catch. Once found mainly in physical-therapy settings, stability balls have become staple pieces of equipment in many health clubs. There are several brand names within the stability-ball category, but they are all essentially the same product.

The most important characteristic of these balls is that they are unstable. Using them challenges your body's neuromuscular system, the communication between your nervous system and your muscles. Your neuromuscular system helps you maintain your balance and your stability as you move or perform a certain exercise. For instance, if you sit down on a stability ball and reach far to one side, your body will immediately get messages that it is out of balance and could potentially fall off. It will automatically adjust to your new position in space, enabling you to remain on the ball.

Stability work is an important component of an integrated program, but how often you do it is up to you. If your goal is to increase muscle size, then you might not want to use the balls often, since you won't be able to use as much weight as when sitting on a machine. However, stability balls are excellent for working on core strength. Many of the workouts in this book give you the option of using stability balls as part of your program.

When you use a stability ball, the size of the ball you want depends on which exercise you're doing. The size of a ball can deceive you if it isn't fully inflated; make sure it doesn't feel squishy when you push into it. When you're doing a bridge with your upper body on the ball, the ball should be big enough so that your thighs are parallel to the floor as you start the exercise. When doing a push-up with your legs on the ball, however, you can make the exercise easier or harder by changing the size of the ball. The bigger the ball, the farther away from the floor your body is, and this makes the exercise more challenging. In the case of a push-up, the difficulty of the exercise also depends on what part of your legs the ball is supporting. If your thighs are resting on the ball, the exercise will be relatively easy. It will be harder if your knees are on top of the ball, and very hard if only your ankles and feet are on the ball. All these variables are explained in the exercise descriptions in chapters 10 through 12, enabling you to make the most efficient choices for your morning workouts.

4

Muscles Into Action

||||||||||||||||||||||||||||||||||||||||||||||||||||||||||||||||||||||||||||||||||||||||||||||||||||||||||||||||||||||||||||||

Y ou are motivated to work out in the morning. You have the workouts in this book, so you're ready to start, right? Well, not quite yet. I know it's tempting to take these routines and either begin your new program with them or use them to enhance the program you are currently doing. But first, you should read this chapter, which covers material that is important for your overall fitness program as well as your morning strength routines. Whether you are relatively new to strength workouts or have been working out for some time, the information here will help you get a safe and effective workout. This chapter covers fundamentals such as good posture, exercise readiness, core integrity, and the basics of healthy joints to help you avoid injury. You will learn some simple exercises and stretches, how to ascertain whether you need them, and ways to incorporate them into your program. You will also learn four different warm-ups you can choose from to make sure your body is ready for the workouts.

Medical Clearance

Before beginning an exercise program, you should determine the necessity for medical clearance. You might need to go to your doctor to make sure it's OK for you to start an exercise program. This might seem counterintuitive. Exercise is good for you; it helps you get and stay healthy—why would anyone need to go to the doctor to be "allowed" to exercise? Actually, there are quite a few reasons.

Basically, exercising is a stress on your body. Exercising makes various systems in your body work harder than they do when you are at rest. Your muscles have to work harder to do the strength training you want. Your heart has to work harder to pump blood to the working muscles, and your blood pressure goes up. If your body cannot handle the stress, that can be harmful. For example, if you have one or more risk factors for heart disease, such as having high blood pressure, being overweight, or having a family history of heart attack or stroke, then your chances of suffering a heart attack increase. When you exercise, your blood pressure increases (which it is supposed to do) as well as your heart rate. If you are out of shape, the stress of exercise can trigger a response such as angina, or pain in the chest upon exertion. This is a sign that you are not getting enough blood and oxygen through your system. In this case a doctor, upon examining you, might tell you to exercise at very low levels for a while or prescribe certain medications.

Regardless of the type of exercise program you use, you need to think about your current health status. What is your family history of disease? Did a blood relative die from a medical condition at an early age? Do you have high blood pressure? What about your cholesterol level? Are you overweight? Do you smoke? All these questions are important, and they are what health and fitness organizations use in creating guidelines for determining whether someone needs to get medical clearance before beginning a new program.

Of course, some exercise programs are more aggressive than others, and for them medical clearance is even more important. If you decide to train for a marathon and you have never run more than one mile in your life, then you should get a medical checkup before you begin. If you want to be a bodybuilder and have never lifted weights, you should probably see a doctor to make sure all your joints can handle the stress. If you just want to start an easy program of walking for 20 minutes each morning, however, and you recently had your yearly checkup and received a clean bill of health, then you are OK to start. In fact, as long as you are in good general health and go to the doctor faithfully for a yearly checkup, it's probably all right to start a moderate exercise program, unless your doctor has told you otherwise or something has happened since your last visit. Use the following questionnaire to determine whether you should get medical clearance before beginning any of the routines in this book.

A classic questionnaire that was developed by the Public Health Agency of Canada and revised in 2002 (see www.csep.ca) is useful in determining whether you need your doctor's OK to begin an exercise program. It is called the PAR-Q (Physical Activity Readiness Questionnaire). This form is presented in figure 4.1.

Physical Activity Readiness
Questionnaire - PAR-Q
(revised 2002)

PAR-Q & YOU

(A Questionnaire for People Aged 15 to 69)

Regular physical activity is fun and healthy, and increasingly more people are starting to become more active every day. Being more active is very safe for most people. However, some people should check with their doctor before they start becoming much more physically active.

If you are planning to become much more physically active than you are now, start by answering the seven questions in the box below. If you are between the ages of 15 and 69, the PAR-Q will tell you if you should check with your doctor before you start. If you are over 69 years of age, and you are not used to being very active, check with your doctor.

Common sense is your best guide when you answer these questions. Please read the questions carefully and answer each one honestly: check YES or NO.

YES	NO		
☐	☐	1.	Has your doctor ever said that you have a heart condition <u>and</u> that you should only do physical activity recommended by a doctor?
☐	☐	2.	Do you feel pain in your chest when you do physical activity?
☐	☐	3.	In the past month, have you had chest pain when you were not doing physical activity?
☐	☐	4.	Do you lose your balance because of dizziness or do you ever lose consciousness?
☐	☐	5.	Do you have a bone or joint problem (for example, back, knee or hip) that could be made worse by a change in your physical activity?
☐	☐	6.	Is your doctor currently prescribing drugs (for example, water pills) for your blood pressure or heart condition?
☐	☐	7.	Do you know of <u>any other reason</u> why you should not do physical activity?

If you answered

YES to one or more questions

Talk with your doctor by phone or in person BEFORE you start becoming much more physically active or BEFORE you have a fitness appraisal. Tell your doctor about the PAR-Q and which questions you answered YES.

- You may be able to do any activity you want — as long as you start slowly and build up gradually. Or, you may need to restrict your activities to those which are safe for you. Talk with your doctor about the kinds of activities you wish to participate in and follow his/her advice.
- Find out which community programs are safe and helpful for you.

NO to all questions

If you answered NO honestly to <u>all</u> PAR-Q questions, you can be reasonably sure that you can:
- start becoming much more physically active – begin slowly and build up gradually. This is the safest and easiest way to go.
- take part in a fitness appraisal – this is an excellent way to determine your basic fitness so that you can plan the best way for you to live actively. It is also highly recommended that you have your blood pressure evaluated. If your reading is over 144/94, talk with your doctor before you start becoming much more physically active.

DELAY BECOMING MUCH MORE ACTIVE:
- if you are not feeling well because of a temporary illness such as a cold or a fever – wait until you feel better; or
- if you are or may be pregnant – talk to your doctor before you start becoming more active.

PLEASE NOTE: If your health changes so that you then answer YES to any of the above questions, tell your fitness or health professional. Ask whether you should change your physical activity plan.

<u>Informed Use of the PAR-Q</u>: The Canadian Society for Exercise Physiology, Health Canada, and their agents assume no liability for persons who undertake physical activity, and if in doubt after completing this questionnaire, consult your doctor prior to physical activity.

No changes permitted. You are encouraged to photocopy the PAR-Q but only if you use the entire form.

NOTE: If the PAR-Q is being given to a person before he or she participates in a physical activity program or a fitness appraisal, this section may be used for legal or administrative purposes.

"I have read, understood and completed this questionnaire. Any questions I had were answered to my full satisfaction."

NAME _____

SIGNATURE _____ DATE _____

SIGNATURE OF PARENT _____ WITNESS _____
or GUARDIAN (for participants under the age of majority)

> **Note: This physical activity clearance is valid for a maximum of 12 months from the date it is completed and becomes invalid if your condition changes so that you would answer YES to any of the seven questions.**

 © Canadian Society for Exercise Physiology   Supported by: Health Santé
Canada Canada

continued on other side...

FIGURE 4.1   PAR-Q form.

Source: Physical Activity Readiness Questionnaire (PAR-Q) © 2002. Reproduced with permission from the Canadian Society for Exercise Physiology. http://www.csep.ca/forms.asp

...continued from other side

PAR-Q & YOU

Physical Activity Readiness
Questionnaire - PAR-Q
(revised 2002)

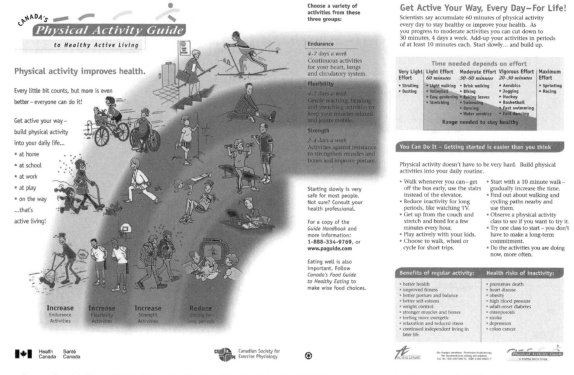

Get Active Your Way, Every Day—For Life!

Scientists say accumulate 60 minutes of physical activity every day to stay healthy or improve your health. As you progress to moderate activities you can cut down to 30 minutes, 4 days a week. Add-up your activities in periods of at least 10 minutes each. Start slowly... and build up.

Time needed depends on effort

Very Light Effort	Light Effort 60 minutes	Moderate Effort 30-60 minutes	Vigorous Effort 20-30 minutes	Maximum Effort
• Strolling • Dusting	• Light walking • Volleyball • Easy gardening • Stretching	• Brisk walking • Biking • Raking leaves • Swimming • Dancing • Water aerobics	• Aerobics • Jogging • Hockey • Basketball • Fast swimming • Fast dancing	• Sprinting • Racing

Range needed to stay healthy

You Can Do It – Getting started is easier than you think

Physical activity doesn't have to be very hard. Build physical activities into your daily routine.

- Walk whenever you can– get off the bus early, use the stairs instead of the elevator.
- Reduce inactivity for long periods, like watching TV.
- Get up from the couch and stretch and bend for a few minutes every hour.
- Play actively with your kids.
- Choose to walk, wheel or cycle for short trips.

- Start with a 10 minute walk– gradually increase the time.
- Find out about walking and cycling paths nearby and use them.
- Observe a physical activity class to see if you want to try it.
- Try one class to start – you don't have to make a long-term commitment.
- Do the activities you are doing now, more often.

Benefits of regular activity:
- better health
- improved fitness
- better posture and balance
- better self-esteem
- weight control
- stronger muscles and bones
- feeling more energetic
- relaxation and reduced stress
- continued independent living in later life

Health risks of inactivity:
- premature death
- heart disease
- obesity
- high blood pressure
- adult-onset diabetes
- osteoporosis
- stroke
- depression
- colon cancer

Source: *Canada's Physical Activity Guide to Healthy Active Living*, Health Canada, 1998 http://www.hc-sc.gc.ca/hppb/paguide/pdf/guideEng.pdf
© Reproduced with permission from the Minister of Public Works and Government Services Canada, 2002.

FITNESS AND HEALTH PROFESSIONALS MAY BE INTERESTED IN THE INFORMATION BELOW:

The following companion forms are available for doctors' use by contacting the Canadian Society for Exercise Physiology (address below):

The **Physical Activity Readiness Medical Examination (PARmed-X)** – to be used by doctors with people who answer YES to one or more questions on the PAR-Q.

The **Physical Activity Readiness Medical Examination for Pregnancy (PARmed-X for Pregnancy)** – to be used by doctors with pregnant patients who wish to become more active.

References:
Arraix, G.A., Wigle, D.T., Mao, Y. (1992). Risk Assessment of Physical Activity and Physical Fitness in the Canada Health Survey Follow-Up Study. **J. Clin. Epidemiol.** 45:4 419-428.
Mottola, M., Wolfe, L.A. (1994). Active Living and Pregnancy, In: A. Quinney, L. Gauvin, T. Wall (eds.), **Toward Active Living: Proceedings of the International Conference on Physical Activity, Fitness and Health**. Champaign, IL: Human Kinetics.
PAR-Q Validation Report, British Columbia Ministry of Health, 1978.
Thomas, S., Reading, J., Shephard, R.J. (1992). Revision of the Physical Activity Readiness Questionnaire (PAR-Q). **Can. J. Spt. Sci.** 17:4 338-345.

To order multiple printed copies of the PAR-Q, please contact the:

Canadian Society for Exercise Physiology
202-185 Somerset Street West
Ottawa, ON K2P 0J2
Tel. 1-877-651-3755 • FAX (613) 234-3565
Online: www.csep.ca

The original PAR-Q was developed by the British Columbia Ministry of Health. It has been revised by an Expert Advisory Committee of the Canadian Society for Exercise Physiology chaired by Dr. N. Gledhill (2002).

Disponible en français sous le titre «Questionnaire sur l'aptitude à l'activité physique - Q-AAP (revisé 2002)».

 © Canadian Society for Exercise Physiology   Supported by: Health Canada Santé Canada

Source: Physical Activity Readiness Questionnaire (PAR-Q) © 2002. Reproduced with permission from the Canadian Society for Exercise Physiology.
http://www.csep.ca/forms.asp

Posture

In fitness terminology, posture indicates how your bones and joints are positioned relative to one another and to gravity. Generally, the ideal posture is *neutral* posture, which is often considered to be the position of your body that is the least stressful. The problem with this definition, however, is that in today's sedentary society, the least stressful posture is slumped forward! Think of neutral posture as your body's natural arrangement and alignment against gravity, but with "natural" meaning the way it was designed to be and not necessarily the way it is now, or how stressful it is to sustain it.

When you have good posture, there is minimal strain on your joints and muscles, because everything is in the right spot. This joint and muscle integrity is discussed in greater detail later in this chapter. Good posture enables you to stand tall, which, as a bonus, contributes to positive self-image and self-esteem.

Good posture during exercise is necessary for targeting the muscles you want and for reducing the chance of injury. Start by looking at your own posture when you are standing. When you look at yourself from the side, your head should be directly above your body, with your ear in line with your shoulder rather than in front of it. It is very common to observe that your head is sticking out in front of your shoulders. When your head is too far forward, the muscles in the back of your neck need to work harder in holding your head up, while the muscles deep in the front of your neck get weak. This imbalance can lead to tightness and discomfort in the neck. Your hip bone should also be lined up with your ear and your shoulder, and your knee and your ankle should be in the same line as well. Both feet should be facing straight ahead, and they should be about hip-width apart. Your shoulders should be pulled back and down without straining. Your abdominal muscles should be engaged, meaning your belly is not sticking out. There should be a slight curve in your low back, and your pelvis should be level. This means that when you put your hands on your hips, you should feel that your front fingers are not much lower than your thumbs in the back. Your hip bones are easy to find in the front; feel for the bony points in the front, and then follow this to the back, right above your butt. With your pelvis level, you can observe the natural curve in your low back, which you should sustain while standing, sitting, or exercising (unless otherwise noted). See figures 4.2 and 4.3 for examples of correct posture.

It's important to assess your own posture and understand what "neutral" is and how to maintain it. I have worked with many clients who finally get the idea of neutral posture while they are standing up, but as soon as they lean over to do single-arm rows, their backs round, their heads stick out, and their necks arch. Although I am stressing good and neutral posture, you *will* need to move out of neutral as part of some exercises. For example, when you sit on the floor to do a rotation exercise for your core, you will be turning to the left and the right with your spine. Your shoulders, however, should still be in the neutral position and not rounding forward. When you do lunges, you will sometimes step to different angles that will take you out of neutral posture. When you come back to the starting position before taking the next step, however, you should more or less be in that neutral position with both feet straight ahead. When you're doing seated exercises, good posture means you are sitting on the bottom of your pelvis, called your sit bones. You should maintain the natural curve in your low back, and keep your shoulders down and back without straining.

Core integrity is important to achieving and maintaining good posture. Your core is the center of your body, or everything besides your arms and your legs. It is where your center of gravity is located and where your power comes from. Having a strong core is vital, because it enables you to transfer loads between your upper and lower body and gives you the support from which to lift weights in your workouts. Core stability and core exercises are discussed in chapter 11. You should become very familiar with engaging these muscles.

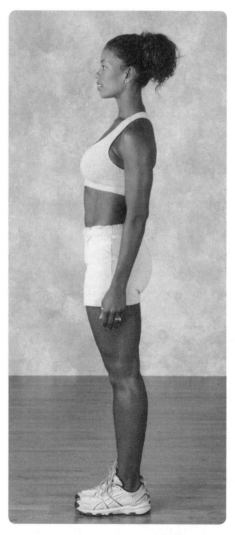

FIGURE 4.2   Correct posture, lateral view.

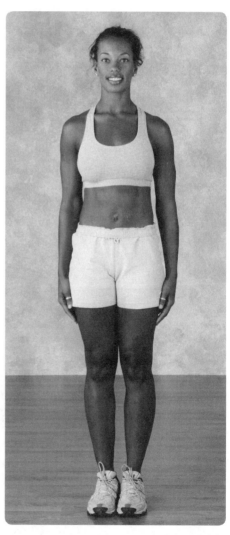

FIGURE 4.3   Correct posture, anterior view.

Joint and Muscle Integrity

Your joints and muscles are also important in maintaining good posture. The integrity of your joints and muscles allows you to lift weights efficiently and safely. If this integrity is impaired, you won't be able to work as hard as you want to in your strength workouts, and you can increase your chance of getting injured. The loss of this integrity is caused by muscle imbalance. Basically, your muscles have an optimal length at which they can function properly. When your muscles are shorter or tighter than optimal, they can pull bones out of alignment. Meanwhile, the opposing muscles on the other side get longer and weaker than optimal, which only exacerbates the imbalanced relationship.

Let's look at a classic example of muscle imbalance and how it contributes to joint discomfort. Many people have a rounded-forward posture at their shoulders. If you look at them from the front, their arms look like they are rotated in so that you see the back of their hands. This posture can be caused by several things, one of which is doing exercises incorrectly. A lat pull-down is a perfect example. As explained in the upper-body exercises in chapter 10, you should pull your shoulders down and back as you pull the bar down. If you allow your shoulders to round forward and up as you pull, your latissimus dorsi muscles, or lats, are not biomechanically able to contract efficiently, because your scapulae, or shoulder blades, are out of position. This constant rounding forward of your shoulders while exercising will cause the anterior fibers of your deltoids, or shoulder muscles, to become shorter and shorter. Chest exercises can also contribute to this posture, since the pectoralis major, or pecs, actually rotate the arm in because of the way the fibers attach to the arm. Often, guys who want to get their chest muscles bigger do too many chest exercises in proportion to the exercises that strengthen the muscles of the upper-middle back. Finally, if you have a job where you work at a computer, this can create a tendency for your shoulders to round forward during the day. The result is that the humerus bone gets pulled forward and up in the shoulder joint by the tight and short muscles of the shoulder, while the opposing muscles of the upper-middle back and the back of the shoulder get long and weak, further encouraging this posture to sustain itself.

To reduce or avoid this posture, be aware of your posture and use good lifting techniques during your workout. It is also important to balance your strength training program by including exercises for the upper-middle back. Finally, looking at the ergonomics of your workstation can help. *Ergonomics* means the physical setup of your desk, computer, phone, and so on, together with the patterns of how you move and hold yourself while you are at work. If you have this posture of forward-rounded shoulders, you should get a headset instead of holding the phone with your ear to your shoulder. You should also make sure that your chair is high enough so that you can rest your arms on the desk comfortably; you should be able to sit up tall and work without having to reach forward with your arms, which puts you into that forward-rounded position.

If you understand some basic information about the desired integrity of some major joints, you will be able to recognize when something is out of alignment. You can then practice some simple techniques, including stretches and exercises that are specifically designed to release tension, to get the muscles around your joints back in balance. This section presents some stretches and exercises that will keep your muscles and joints flexible, healthy, and ready for action. After reading about potential imbalances around your ankle, hip, and shoulder, you can determine for yourself whether you need to use the suggested techniques. For example, if you sat at a desk all day and then looked at your posture and saw that your shoulders were rounded forward, then you should incorporate the reach, roll, and lift exercise into your exercise routine, or even do it every day. Or if you try the calf stretch and feel a lot of tightness, that means you need to do the stretch often. If you find that after several weeks your calves don't feel as tight anymore, then you can just do the stretch every few weeks. This is called *maintaining the integrity*.

Foot and Ankle

Foot and ankle integrity is important in your strength workouts, since many of the exercises are done while standing or moving on your feet. When you have imbalances around your foot and ankle, your foot can roll too much in one direction or the other and make you feel unstable.

Many people live with aches and pains around the foot and ankle that are due to muscle imbalances. If your arch is either flatter or higher than it should be, muscles around your foot and up around your shin get either tighter or longer than they should be, and that can lead to knee discomfort. This can go even farther up the chain of your body to the hip and eventually the low back. Such discomfort will make your exercises uncomfortable and will be detrimental to your strength workouts.

Learning what "neutral" is at the foot and ankle will help prevent aches and pains and potential injuries. To get to neutral, put on a pair of shorts and stand barefoot while facing a mirror with your feet straight ahead and hip-width apart. Do your feet flatten at the arch? Do you have very high arches so that you feel you are putting all your weight on the outside of your feet? Looking at your legs and feet, rotate your thighs and entire legs to the inside and then to the outside. When you turn them in, you should see that your arches flatten out (pronation), and when you turn them out, you should see that your arches lift up (supination). Find the halfway point, and then hold it. This is a good neutral position. Achieving this position is what you pay lots of money for when you buy sneakers; they have material in the shoes to give you support in the appropriate places to maintain a neutral arch position. As you walk, it is natural for your foot and ankle to pronate as you place your foot on the ground, and as you push off for the next step, it is natural to supinate. Many people, however, overpronate so that their arch collapses and doesn't supinate, causing tension up the leg.

If you observe that the arches of your feet collapse or flatten very easily, you might want to go to a podiatrist to see if orthotics are appropriate for you. If you feel that you can lift up your arch but need lots of focus to maintain that position, you should do the single-leg heel raise with foot turned in with dumbbell, described in chapter 12 (page 213). Doing it with your foot turned in focuses on the muscles that help with arch integrity, especially the tibialis posterior, which is a deep calf muscle that attaches to the bottom of your foot. As it contracts, it shortens the fibers of your arch, helping to keep your foot less pronated. If you try this exercise and really feel it deep in your calf as well as in your arch on the bottom of your foot, then you should do two sets of 15 to 25 repetitions of this exercise every time you work out. When you notice that the integrity of your arch has improved, you can do the exercise less frequently to maintain the integrity.

If you have a higher-than-normal arch and walk on the outsides of your feet, you should also find out whether orthotics might be appropriate for you. The muscles around your foot and ankle can be tight and short. You could also benefit from calf stretches (discussed a bit further on) and self-myofascial release on the muscles on the lateral side (outside) of your leg. Self-myofascial release, or SMR, is a technique that releases tension in your muscle fibers. This tension is caused by the muscle imbalances described earlier in this chapter. Actin and myosin, the protein filaments that contract as you exercise, do not glide across each other efficiently when one muscle is out of balance, because the filaments are basically out of position. Then, the fascia (tissue that wraps around each muscle) tightens up too. You can feel this tightness when you press on the area, like knots along your muscle fibers.

SMR is similar to when someone gives you a friendly massage and you feel tension in a very specific spot and tell them to massage right there. Pressure point massage is based on this principle. When you do SMR and use a foam roller or soft ball like a tennis ball to put pressure on these knots, you can help them neurologically release and feel much less tight. Styrofoam rollers come in different sizes. For the SMR, get one that is full size (3 feet or .9 meter long) and is a full round roller. You can buy them from fitness equipment brochures. One Web site that sells rollers as well as other fitness equipment is www.performbetter.com.

To do SMR on your calf muscles, start by sitting on the floor with the roller beneath your right calf with its ends pointing to either side. Slowly move your body so that the roller glides up and down along the bottom of your calf. You can increase the pressure by putting your left leg on top of your right. Don't worry about finding the knots—they will find you! Turn your leg so that the outside of your calf is on the roller (see figure 4.4), then the inside. When you feel tension, try to stay on that point, or as close to it as possible, and just breathe for 20 to 30 seconds. You will feel the pressure decrease and more blood flowing to that area. Doing this at the beginning of your workout can help increase blood and oxygen flow and reduce tension. As was discussed in chapter 2, you can also use tennis balls in a sock to get the same effect.

Another way to help alleviate the tension from a high arch and tight muscles on the outside of your leg is to do the calf stretch. Stand facing a wall or chair with

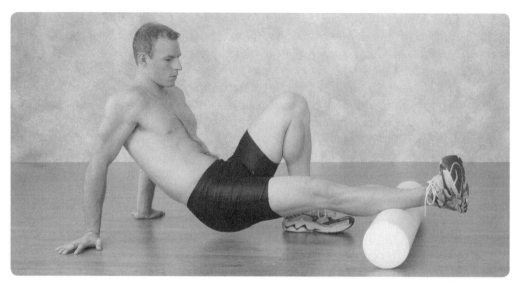

FIGURE 4.4   SMR for calf.

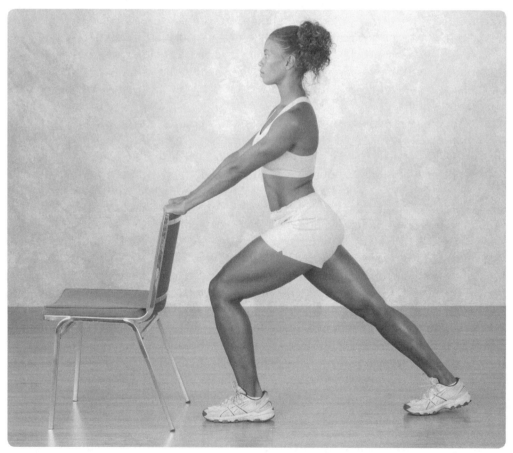

FIGURE 4.5   Calf stretch.

your right leg about three feet (about one meter) behind the left. Keeping your hip bones still, turn your whole right leg in. Push your right heel into the floor while leaning forward with your whole body (see figure 4.5 on the previous page). If you need this stretch, you will feel it on the outside of your calf, down your leg, and into your foot. You can try this same stretch with your leg turned out instead of in, and see if you feel that more. If you really feel your calf stretching in either direction, do this as part of your warm-up before each workout, and more often if you can. If you notice a big stretch, it wouldn't be a bad idea to do this for a few minutes every day. If you find that the tightness lessens over time, you can just use the stretch when you feel you particularly need it—if you're sore after a hard workout, for example, or a long run.

Hip

Your actual hip joint is the point at which your femur, or thighbone, meets the acetabulum of your pelvis, which is your hip socket. In general, though, when we refer to your hips we mean your entire pelvis. Hip integrity is important because it helps your low back. When the muscles of your hip are strong and in balance, your low back does not have to work as hard as it would otherwise. Your habits can affect this. For example, when you bend down to pick something up from the floor, you should flex, or bend, at the hips and push your butt back. This allows your glutes, or butt muscles, to work efficiently. If you don't do this, you will flex from your spine, which puts undue stress on the ligaments along the spine.

All the muscles that start at, attach to, or cross through your pelvis work as a team. The hip flexors are responsible for tilting your pelvis anteriorly, increasing the curve in your low back. These are balanced by the glutes, abs, and hamstrings, which tilt your pelvis posteriorly, decreasing the curve in your low back. When all these muscles are of the proper length, your pelvis is neutral and level as described earlier in this chapter. Your hamstring muscles are also important in maintaining the integrity of your pelvis, as well as your SI, or sacroiliac, joint, which is where the two halves of your pelvis meet your sacrum, the triangle-shaped bone at the bottom of your spine. This integrity is also crucial to the health of your low back.

Sitting for long periods of time can affect the overall integrity of your hips and your spine. Even in good posture, your hip flexors would be in a constantly shortened position, which is discussed a bit later. Let's look at another scenario that happens all too often in which the hamstrings contribute to poor hip integrity. There are three hamstring muscles; they start at the bottom of your pelvis, go down the back of your thigh, and attach below the knee to the tibia and fibula, the bones of the lower leg. Poor sitting posture can lead to your hamstrings becoming tight and short at the hip. This pulls your pelvis into a posterior tilt, decreasing the natural curve in your low back—think of sitting at your desk with your butt tucked under and your low back flexed forward. Because your spine is flexed forward, the muscles that run along your spine get longer than they should be. Your muscles' response is to get tight in an effort to protect your spine in this undesirable position. Now your back starts to hurt, but it isn't actually a back problem!

To see if your hamstrings are short and tight, stand with your feet hip-width apart and straight ahead. Put your right heel on an elevated surface such as a step, and keep your leg straight at the knee (see figure 4.6a). Keeping the natural curve in your low back, lean forward from your hip (see figure 4.6b). If you feel a stretch in the hamstrings, along the back of your thigh, before you lean far enough forward to get your upper body perpendicular to the leg you are stretching, you need to stretch your hamstrings by holding this position for 20 to 30 seconds.

Let's look at another example, where muscles around your hip can create knee discomfort. You might notice when you do a squat or leg press that your thighs tend to cave in. This is often because the muscles on the lateral side (outside) of your hip are weaker than they should be. This is your gluteus medius muscle. It is under the larger gluteus maximus muscle, and one of its jobs is to prevent your femur, or thighbone, from rolling in too much when you walk or run. Every time you step, your leg rolls in (pronates); this is normal. If this muscle is weak, how-

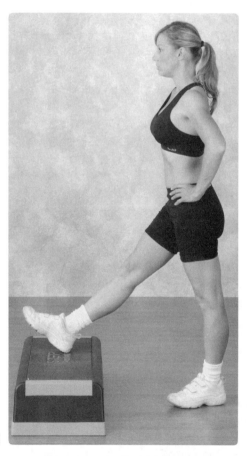 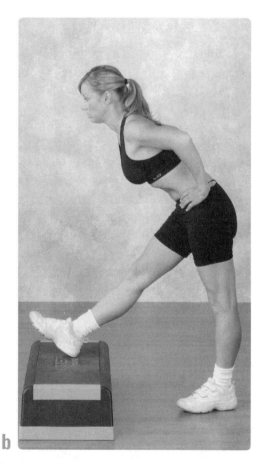

FIGURE 4.6   Hamstring stretch: *(a)* start position, *(b)* end position.

ever, your thigh will roll in too much and stay rolled in. Your patella, or kneecap, is now out of position, increasing the pressure around it. This can lead to tension in your iliotibial band, which is explained shortly. This is not fundamentally a knee problem! To solve it, you need to strengthen your gluteus medius. The band walking exercise in chapter 12 (see page 211) is perfect for targeting this muscle. If you are someone whose thighs do tend to collapse in, then you will feel that this exercise is challenging as soon as you start doing it. Do the exercise before every workout until you notice that it's easier for you to keep your legs hip-width apart when you squat or lunge. At that point, you can just use it once in a while to maintain the integrity.

Your iliotibial band, also called the IT band, is a fibrous band of tissue that runs from the side of your hip and down along the outside of your thigh to your tibia bone, below your knee. Repetitive motions such as running can irritate the attachment at the outside of the knee, since running requires constant flexing or bending at the knee and hip, with the necessary internal rotation of your femur, as discussed previously. If your gluteus medius is weaker than it needs to be, and your thigh rolls in too much, your IT band gets short and therefore tight where it attaches outside the knee at the tibia, again causing knee discomfort. It is difficult to stretch the IT band because of the tissue it is composed of, but doing the self-myofascial release is very beneficial.

To do SMR on your IT band, sit on the floor with the outside of your right thigh on the roller. Put your left leg across your right leg and your left foot on the floor for more stability, and hold yourself up with your upper body (see figure 4.7). Roll up and down until you feel knots along the IT band. Hold the position on any tender spot for 20 to 30 seconds. Then switch to the left leg.

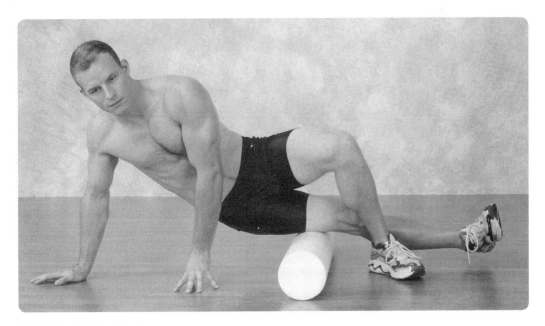

FIGURE 4.7   SMR for IT band.

As stated earlier, poor posture when sitting can lead to tight and short hamstrings if you slouch forward and constantly round your back. Poor posture can also lead to tight and short hip flexors. Your hip flexor muscles are also important in maintaining hip integrity. The psoas attaches to the front of your spine, and the iliacus to the inside of your pelvis. Together, they attach to the front of your femur. The rectus femoris, one of the quadriceps, also helps flex the hip. Even sitting in good posture shortens these muscles, since you are flexed at the hip, with your low back essentially closer to your thigh than when standing. As these muscles get tighter and shorter, they can tilt your pelvis anteriorly, increasing the curve in your low back. The problem can be exacerbated by weak abs and glutes, since they are supposed to counterbalance the action of the hip flexors. Since the psoas attaches to the front of the vertebrae, or bones of the spine, it creates tension on them. This leads to discomfort of the spine, or low back pain. If when you examined your own posture as explained earlier you observed that your pelvis seems to be tilted forward, you will probably really feel the hip flexor stretch that follows.

To do the hip flexor stretch, stand with your feet about hip-width apart and bring your right leg about three feet (about one meter) behind your left. Keeping your hip bones neutral, turn your right leg in, keeping your heel on the floor. Contract your abdominal muscles and your glutes to flatten out your low back and get into more of a posterior pelvic tilt. Reach your right arm up toward the ceiling, and then reach it up and over to the left (see figure 4.8). You should feel a nice stretch in the front of your thigh and up into your abs. Hold for 20 seconds. If you feel a strong stretch, you should do this before every workout. When you notice that the stretch feels less intense, you can just use it every once in a while.

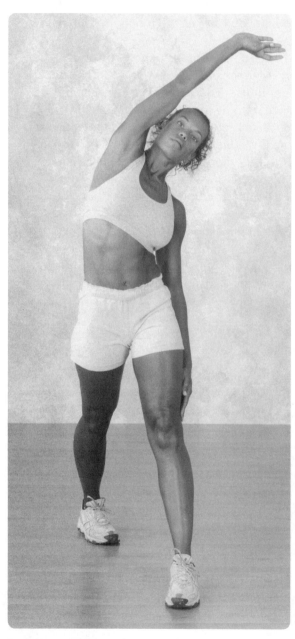

FIGURE 4.8 Hip flexor stretch.

If your hip flexors are tight and short and your pelvis is in an anterior tilt, it is more difficult for your gluteus maximus to work, since it is now in a lengthened position from which it's harder to contract. You can demonstrate this for yourself with the following quick example. Stand with your feet hip-width apart. Stick your butt out, increasing the curve in your low back as much as possible. Now try to contract your glutes (i.e., squeeze your butt). You might find it difficult or even impossible, because it puts the muscle in a biomechanically difficult position from which to contract. As the chain reaction continues, the piriformis muscle tries to work too soon, contracting out of sequence and causing more tension in this area. Your piriformis is a deep external hip rotator located underneath your gluteus maximus. If this muscle gets tight or inflamed, it can aggravate the sciatic nerve, which leads to tension or tingly feelings down the back of your leg. Doing SMR for the piriformis is important if you feel this discomfort or notice that your hip flexors are tight and short. You will also need to strengthen your glutes with the bridges explained in chapter 12 and your deep core stabilizers as explained in chapter 11.

To do the SMR for the piriformis, sit right on top of the roller, putting your arms behind you and leaning back onto your hands. Turn over a bit to your right and move the roller around under your gluteus maximus on that side (see figure 4.9). When you feel a tender spot, stay at that spot for 20 to 30 seconds. Do the same on the left side.

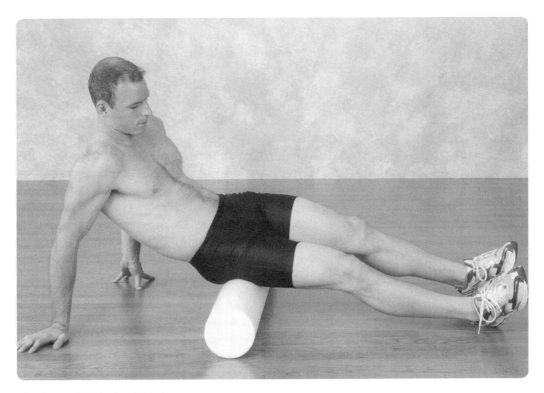

FIGURE 4.9　SMR for the piriformis.

Shoulder

Your shoulder girdle is made up of your shoulder blades, or scapulae, in the back; your collarbones, or clavicles, in the front; and your sternum, or breastbone, also in the front. For general good posture, try to keep your scapulae down and back without straining. Your shoulder joint is made up of your upper arm, or humerus, in its socket, which is part of the scapula. Your humerus has a large range of motion in which it can move, but there is not much room on top of it because of the other muscles and tendons that cross through that area. When you sit in poor posture with your shoulders rounded forward or lift weights using poor form, it can lead to your humerus being too forward and too high in your shoulder joint. With your humerus out of alignment, the tendons on top can get pinched, causing discomfort when you lift up your arm.

When you observe your posture from the side, does your shoulder look like it is internally rotated (rounded forward)? Can you pull your shoulders back without straining? Is it difficult for you to hold them in this good posture over an extended period of time, like when you're sitting at your desk, for example? You should always hold your shoulders down and back without straining. This is especially crucial when lifting weights; adding more stress to the area makes it all the more important to keep the bones in the correct position.

Another point to keep in mind is that when you do an exercise like a row, your shoulder blades should move along with the motions of your arms. It shouldn't be a big movement, just a subtle rhythm of your shoulder girdle and your shoulder joint. When your shoulder girdle moves with your arm, there will be enough room for your humerus to move around without pinching any muscles or tendons.

If you see that your shoulders are rounded forward and you feel that it is difficult to keep them back and down in good posture, you should do more exercises for the muscles on the back side of your torso in proportion to the exercises you do for the front side. In general, that means more pulling exercises than pushing exercises—more rows than chest presses, for example.

One exercise that will help keep your shoulders healthy is the reach, roll, and lift (see page 165). This exercise is integrated, meaning that it gets several parts of your body working together to put you in a certain position. It's designed to get your lower trapezius muscles working, which helps you pull your shoulder blades down and thereby releases the upper trapezius, which is the opposite muscle group. If you find the exercise difficult, you should do one set of 25 lifts before every workout. When you notice that it has become easier to keep your shoulders back and down and your posture is better, then you can just do the exercise once in a while for maintenance.

You should also determine whether the muscles in the front are short and tight. This could be because of rounding the shoulders described previously or doing too many chest exercises compared with exercises done for the upper-middle back muscles. Stand with your right side next to a doorjamb or at a place where a wall turns a corner. Hold your right arm up and out to the side, with your elbow a little below shoulder height, forming a right angle at your elbow. Put your right arm against the wall in this position so that most of it is touching the surface. Gently lean forward (into the doorway or past the corner) and rotate your upper body slightly to the left. Hold for 20 seconds. You should feel a stretch along the front of your body, either in your chest (pec muscles) or in the front of your shoulders. If you feel a big stretch, you should do this before every workout until it gets easier. If you feel a relatively slight stretch, then you only need to do this once in a while or as needed, like if you are sore after doing plyometric push-ups, for example.

Warming Up

The last step before getting into your workout is warming up. Your workout should always begin with a warm-up. If you have determined that you need some of the stretches, self-myofascial release, or exercises described earlier in this chapter, then this is the time to do those also.

Warming up is more important before a morning workout than before a workout later in the day. During the night as you sleep, your muscles and joints need less blood and oxygen than when you are up and moving around, and so they cool down. Warming up in the morning before you exercise will help to increase your blood flow, elevate your body temperature, and get your muscles and joints warm and ready for the workout you've decided to do that day. Doing so is very important because cold muscles and joints don't react to stress as quickly and effectively as warm ones, which means they can get injured more easily.

Warming up also prepares your mind to focus on the workout ahead. What exercises are you going to do today? Is there any particularly challenging exercise that will demand your utmost concentration? It also allows you to take an inventory of how your body is feeling. As you go through the movements in these warm-ups, you'll have the opportunity to notice any stiffness you may have from the previous workout and to make some last-minute changes if necessary. For example, if your last workout was more challenging for your legs than you are used to and they feel sore, you might decide to pick a shorter workout today or do a workout that focuses on your arms.

There are lots of options for you when you're deciding what form your warm-up will take. At home or outside you can walk in place or do jumping jacks. In the gym, you can use one of the numerous pieces of cardiovascular equipment, such as a treadmill, bicycle, or elliptical machine. You should set the machine at a low level of resistance or intensity. When you break a sweat or your breathing becomes a little labored and your heart rate has increased, which usually takes about five minutes, you are ready to start.

This section offers you four other choices in addition to the traditional cardio warm-up just described. Integrated training is described in chapter 5, but basically, these warm-ups accord with the idea of integrated workouts by having you move your body in all three planes of motion—you will move forward and back, move side to side, and rotate. This will "fire up" your neuromuscular system—the connection between your muscles and your nerves that helps you move efficiently and in a coordinated manner. The first is a core warm-up. The second is based on several components: your body weight; moving in different directions; and the reach, roll, and lift exercise to keep your shoulders healthy. The third warm-up uses a stability ball. The fourth uses a medicine ball and is based on squats and diagonal patterns. Besides being great choices for warm-ups, any or all of these can also be done as workouts at home, outside, or at the gym.

Core Warm-Up

This warm-up focuses on the muscles of your core, as well as challenges the rest of your body. If you want to get your midsection tighter, this is a great choice for a warm-up. You could also do this as a workout at home, doing the entire series four or five times. This is a great "makeup" routine if you've missed your Pilates class! Since your core is neurologically wired to transfer forces between your upper and lower body, this warm-up helps your body get neurologically prepared for your strength training after you've been sleeping all night. This helps you even more if you are going to do a workout with heavy weights, since your core helps you stay stable from the inside out, making it easier to lift the weight. All these exercises are explained in chapter 11. Do the entire sequence twice.

- Toe tap: Page 169. 10 reps each side.
- Seated rotation with no extra resistance: This is a modification of the seated rotation with dumbbell. Since it is a warm-up, you don't need the extra resistance. Page 179. 10 reps each side.
- Prone hold on forearms: Page 174. 10 seconds.
- Lateral hold on forearm: Page 176. 10 seconds.
- Back extension: Page 185. 10 reps.
- Prone hold on hands: Page 175. 10 seconds.
- Lateral hold with straight arm: Page 177. 10 seconds.

Body-Weight Warm-Up

This workout has several purposes, so if you want a warm-up with a little of everything, you will like this choice. It moves your whole body along the three planes of motion, which basically means in all different directions. This is great for getting your neuromuscular system going, because it means your brain has to work a little harder than just moving forward and back or doing a traditional warm-up on a bicycle, for example. In this warm-up you will do the reach, roll, and lift, which is a corrective exercise for your shoulders and upper-body posture. There is also a spine stabilization exercise, the opposite arm/leg reach, and clock lunges, which will help you warm up all the muscles around your hips. Do the entire sequence twice.

- Forward lunge with lateral flexion: With your arms up, step forward with your right leg and flex or bend your upper body to the right at the same time. Five to each side.
- Rotation lunge with no dumbbells: Page 204. Limit your range of motion by not stepping as far and deep as you normally would. One time clockwise, one time counterclockwise.
- Push-up: Page 146. Again, limit your range of motion. 5 reps.
- Reach, roll, and lift: Page 165. 5 reps.
- Opposite arm/leg reach: Page 173. 5 reps.
- Single-leg bridge on floor: Page 210. 10 reps.

Full-Body Warm-Up With Stability Ball

This warm-up is perfect for you if you like using the stability ball. Some people simply love the stability ball, and this warm-up is a great excuse to use it! This warm-up challenges your core muscles and your balance and stability. In general, using a stability ball automatically puts a greater demand on your core muscles than the same exercise off the ball would do. When you do the bridges, for example, your core muscles have to work to hold you still on the ball—much more demanding than doing a bridge on the floor. Using the stability ball means your neuromuscular system will be challenged. This is explained in more detail in chapter 5. It is important to incorporate this variable at least now and then so that your coordination and balance improve along with your strength and size. Do the entire sequence of the following exercises two or three times.

- Single-leg squat with opposite-arm reach: Page 197. Use a very limited range of motion for the squat.
- Bridge with lower body on stability ball: Page 208. 10 reps.
- Bridge with upper body on stability ball: Page 209. 10 reps.
- Lat roll-out on stability ball: Page 144. Five reps with limited range of motion.
- Push-up with legs on stability ball: Page 149. Use a limited range of motion. 10 reps.

Full-Body Warm-Up With Medicine Ball

Use a medicine ball that weighs about two to four pounds (0.9–1.8 kilograms). Just make sure it doesn't feel too heavy—if it does, start by using a water bottle and work your way up to a medicine ball. What you are aiming for is simply a feeling of resistance so that holding it out in front of you will make you engage your core muscles. Stand with your feet hip-width apart and hold the ball in front of you. Your arms should be fairly straight, but keep your elbows soft. Squat down and then stand up, bringing the ball overhead as you stand (see figure 4.10). Keep your core muscles engaged the entire time, but try to pull them in slightly more as you change direction from going down to up. After eight repetitions, change the angle. Squat down toward your left foot, keeping both feet on the floor but allowing your body to turn gently to the left, and bring the ball overhead, above your right shoulder, making a diagonal line across your body. Think of squatting down to pick up a bag that is on the floor by your left foot. It is not heavy enough for you to have to turn your whole body, just turn as you squat down, with your right knee moving in as you squat and turn to the left (see figure 4.11). You can make these movements more challenging by pretending that you are going to throw the ball over your shoulder as you stand up. Keep your arms relatively straight with your elbows soft. You will immediately notice how your abs and entire core have to work to control the movement. Do eight reps and then switch sides, bringing the ball from the right foot up and over the left shoulder. The last step is to stand and rotate your entire body from side to side while holding the medicine ball out in front of your body with your arms straight but not locked at the elbows. Keep your feet on the ground as you rotate to your right and then to your left (see figure 4.12).

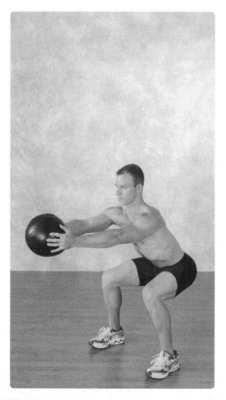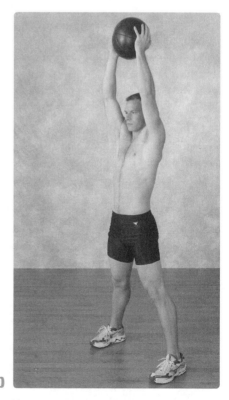

FIGURE 4.10   Vertical move: *(a)* starting position, *(b)* end position.

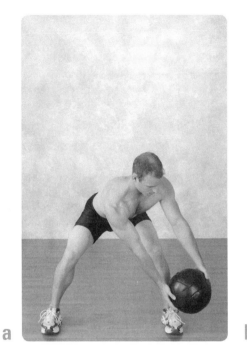
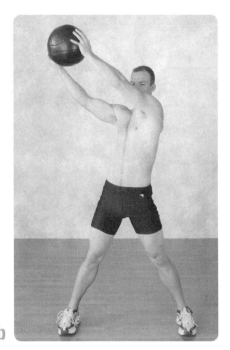

FIGURE 4.11   Diagonal move: *(a)* starting position, *(b)* end position.

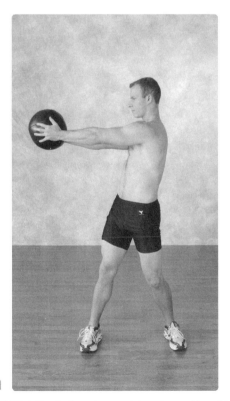
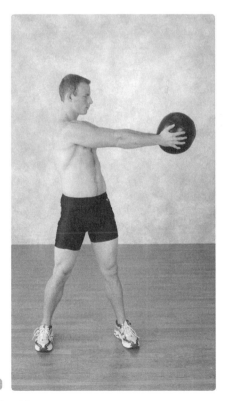

FIGURE 4.12   Horizontal move: *(a)* starting position, *(b)* end position.

5

Developing Your Training Program

||||||||||||||||||||||||||||||||||||||||||||||||||||||||||||||||||||||||||||||||||||||||||||||||||||||||||||||

Since you are a morning exerciser, you have already made your exercise program a priority (or else you wouldn't give up those extra z's!). Now you need to decide how to be as efficient as possible with your time and what the goals of your program will be. Keep in mind that there is no one program that is best for everyone. What is important, rather, is determining what kind of training program is right for *you*. Your morning strength program belongs to you and should be designed to fit your individual needs.

This chapter will help you make the best choices for setting goals, tracking your progress, and making sure the workouts you perform are effective and efficient. It will help you establish goals, which are the foundation of any successful program, and then show you how to pick the best routines from chapters 6 through 9 in order to reach them. It will also help you understand why you might want to make changes to the workouts in this book and how to do so. The concept of integrated training, which means challenging more variables than simply the amount of weight you lift, will be presented. Sample logs show you how to keep track of your workouts as well as your diet and energy levels. Last but not least, the issues of rest and overtraining are discussed so that you can avoid unnecessary setbacks and reap the rewards of all your morning workout efforts.

Setting Workout Goals

Many people don't set any goals at all for their fitness programs. This is a big mistake! Goal setting helps you set a path for your workouts and enables you to be clear as to why you are lifting the weight you are lifting and why you are doing a particular workout. It is very important for your goals to be realistic, specific, and measurable. New Year's resolutions are usually perfect examples of goals that are not. People drink too much and then say they are going to start exercising or get in shape. Having the intention is good, but simply saying it is not enough. You need to go one step further and set goals that are realistic, specific, and measurable. Here are the components of effective goal setting:

- **Realistic.** Realistic means the goal is practical—for your lifestyle and for your commitment level. This makes it more likely that you will follow through with it. You might have gone through this thought process already in deciding to be a morning exerciser. Maybe you tried going to the gym after work, and over time you realized that your schedule always seemed to get in the way or that you preferred to go to happy hour instead of the gym. When it became clear to you that exercising in the morning meant there were fewer things to get in your way, you adjusted accordingly. This is being realistic. Making it easier to be consistent increases your chances of success. Setting a realistic goal for your strength workouts is crucial. Do you want to get bigger? If so, how many days per week can you commit to your workouts? How much time can you take in the morning for your workout? If you want to add muscle to your whole body but you're only willing to commit to two workouts each week and only 30 minutes each time, you are not being realistic with yourself, because that is not enough time to reach that goal.

- **Specific.** The more specific you are, the better you are able to determine which actions are necessary to reach your goals. For example, if you have a vague idea that you want to get stronger but don't specify exactly what you have in mind—which might, if you really pinpointed it, be getting stronger in body-weight exercises such as push-ups and chin-ups—you could pick a routine that leads you in a different direction, such as one that focuses on using machines. It's not that you wouldn't get any benefit from those exercises, of course. It's just that your body is incredibly good at getting better at precisely the movement or exercise you do. In this example, the more you gear your workouts to the body-weight exercises, the better you will be at them. And in general, the more specific your goals, the more likely you'll know exactly what you need to do to meet them.

- **Measurable.** Setting a measurable goal means making a plan based on specific behaviors and establishing criteria by which you can tell how much progress you're making toward your goal—and when you have met it! You need to describe the precise actions you will take to reach your goal. For example, if you decide that you want to get good at doing push-ups, that's a goal, but what exactly are you going to do to get to that goal? How many push-ups do you want to be able to do and by when? Perhaps you decide that your goal is to do 20 perfect push-ups and you want to be able to do that by your 40th birthday, which is in two months. To reach your goal, it would be helpful to decide that every morning, whether you work out or not, you are going to do as many push-ups as you can in good form, and at the end of each week you will be able to complete two more push-ups than the week before. You now have a goal by which you can measure your progress, daily and weekly.

So, back to you. Before you begin a workout routine, it's important to know what you want in the end. Ask yourself some questions: What is the purpose of your morning strength workouts? Think about your lifestyle, what you want to get out of the workouts, and how much time you can dedicate to them in the morning. Once you figure these things out and set yourself a goal, it's time to look at how you can start working toward it. How much should you lift, and how many repetitions should you do? The following sections discuss the different types of training that you can use to meet your goals—whether those goals involve strength, size, endurance, power, or general health and fitness—and why you might choose a certain type of training over another. The following sections also explain the more nitty-gritty details you need to consider, such as the number of sets and repetitions you need to do during each workout based on your goal. Once you figure out the type of training you need to do to work toward your goal, you can choose from a number of workouts in part II of this book that are geared to that purpose. In the workouts in this book, you'll see that often the same exercise can be done for different goals but the number of sets you do, the number of repetitions you do, and the weight you need to lift will be different. After you embark on your plan, you should monitor how things go to see if your commitment of time and workouts per week are enough to get the desired results. If not, you will need to either increase the number of workouts you do each week or lengthen the routines. Or you might have to adjust your goals if you are having difficulty reaching them. Remember, that's the realistic part of proper goal setting.

Strength

Is your main goal to increase your strength? What does being stronger mean to you? Why exactly do you want to be stronger than you are now? Many people simply like the general feeling of well-being that comes with increased strength. Exercise makes your body feel better in general, and it is motivating to see that you can lift heavier weight over time. Perhaps increasing your strength is important to you because you feel weak when performing certain daily tasks. Maybe you went on a vacation and noticed that you had a hard time getting your luggage into the overhead bin on the airplane. Having the strength to do things during your day without excess strain or fatigue is crucial to a healthier life. Whatever your reason is, workouts designed to increase strength are great for boosting your general feeling of well-being.

Have you ever noticed after doing an exercise a few times that suddenly you were noticeably stronger? This is caused by the neural adaptations of strength training.

What this means is that once your body's nerves and muscles have "learned" how to do the exercise, they can handle more weight relatively quickly. Learning what is called a *motor pattern* means developing and then perfecting the exact movement with the appropriate energy, like getting the knack of riding a bike. Once you know how to do it, you perfect it by exercising consistently over a long period.

To increase your strength, you need to train your whole body at least two times per week. You don't need to do many repetitions to increase strength—only about 8 to 10, which fits perfectly into a morning routine when the minutes might be clicking away faster than you want. As was just explained, strength is largely neurological, and in fact you don't need to be muscularly big to be strong. The resistance does need to be challenging for the number of reps you do, however. In other words, if you are capable of lifting the weight 15 times but you stop at 8, you are not going to get the results you want. With the optimal amount of weight, you will reach momentary muscular failure by the time you get to 10 repetitions. If you find you can lift the weight more than 10 times in good form, you should increase the weight next time. Increase weight for lower-body exercises by about 10 percent at a time and weight for upper-body exercises by about 5 percent at a time. This is just a general guideline, though. If you increase the weight by 10 percent and can only do five reps, then make it lighter. You will get better at "feeling" whether the weight is too heavy or too light as you continue with your routines.

When you work out, you should lift the weight relatively slowly, using a count of about two seconds to lift the weight, one second to hold it in the lifted position, and then about four seconds to lower the weight. Since the weight you are lifting is relatively heavy, use plenty of control as you perform each movement. For example, when you're doing the row with the dumbbell and you lower the weight, be sure that your arm doesn't just "fall" toward the floor, allowing your elbow to straighten out abruptly; your motion should be slow and deliberate. You should always be in control of the movement in weightlifting, but this is especially important in the morning, since your body is not as warm as it would be later in the day. When lifting relatively heavy weights, keep the range of motion on the conservative side—that makes it easier for you to control the movement and lessens the stress on your joints. Using these guidelines will ensure that you get a safe and effective workout.

Size

Maybe you have determined that you want to add size to your body and look more muscular. Why do you want more muscle? Is it because you think it will make you look better? Many people think that wanting to get bigger is a superficial goal, since it is mainly about aesthetics. There is nothing wrong with an aesthetic goal. There's no doubt that if you feel better about how you look, your self-esteem improves. This can be very motivating for you and even give you the confidence to address other areas of your life that you want to change.

Are there certain muscles that you want to concentrate on, or do you want to be bigger in general? To get bigger, you need to devote relatively more time and energy to working out than you do if your goal is to increase strength. You need more food and more stimulus, which means a greater volume of training—more reps and more workouts. Ask any bodybuilder how hard it is to add muscle size—the answer will be "Very hard!" The first thing you need to understand is that the degree to which you can build muscle is genetically determined. So blame your parents! Some people have more of the fast-twitch muscle fibers that are conducive to getting bigger. Others have more of the slow-twitch fibers that cannot produce as much force but *can sustain* contractions over and over again, which makes them more conducive to lighter weights and more reps. Besides having the genetic potential to build muscle, you have to eat enough, and you have to put a lot of time into your weightlifting program. When working out to increase size, be sure to keep these factors in mind as you set your goals.

If you want to add muscle, you need to do the 60-minute routines at least three days each week. If you can't spare that much time in the morning, there are ways to manipulate the routines in this book. You could do 30- or 45-minute routines and focus on either your upper body or your lower body for each workout—just combine the upper-body exercises from two different routines on one day, and combine the lower-body exercises from both routines the next day you work out. Or you can go through chapter 10 and pick upper-body exercises to make up your own routine, and then next time go through chapter 12 to find exercises for your lower body.

If your goal involves adding muscle mass, you need to do more repetitions than when working for strength. Because of the increased number of repetitions necessary to stimulate the muscle fibers that grow so they reach the state called muscle hypertrophy, you need to use a lighter weight than when training for strength. You need to do more sets during each workout, however, and target the muscles more times each week. This means you are increasing the volume of your training.

Pick a weight that you can lift between 10 and 15 times. Ten reps is the low end of the range for building size, and it is also the high end of the range for building strength; there is a slight overlap on the continuum. In any case, make sure that the weight is challenging enough that you cannot lift it more than 15 times. Again, to find your ideal weight for size workouts, increase the weight for lower-body exercises in increments of about 10 percent, and increase the weight for upper-body exercises in increments of about 5 percent. If something feels much too heavy or much too light, adjust accordingly. Working out in the morning before work or other commitments means that you need to be efficient. Picking the correct weight is important for getting the most out of each repetition and each set of every exercise. When you work out, you should lift the weight relatively slowly, using a count of about two seconds to lift the weight, one second to hold it in the lifted position, and four seconds to lower the weight.

Endurance

Do you want to use your strength program to develop muscular endurance? Muscular endurance is related to muscular strength, but endurance means being able to keep doing a certain exercise or movement over a long period of time. In daily life, it means not getting exhausted from picking up your kid over and over again. Maybe you remember noticing the last time you moved how fatigued you got from carrying boxes all day.

Endurance training is what you need when you are required to be strong doing something for a long period. Endurance exercises are good if you want to be a better long-distance cyclist, because they improve your muscles' ability to take in and use oxygen over the course of a long ride. If you are a cyclist, you also need power to get up the steep hills. How about long-distance running? Runners are notorious for neglecting to do strength exercises, especially for their upper bodies. In fact, your upper body is very important in long-distance running, because it is working to counterbalance the movement of your legs. You also have to hold up your arms as you run. Endurance training can be useful for a variety of goals.

To increase your muscular endurance, try to get in at least two workouts per week—the longer workouts, if possible. For the endurance routines, pick a weight that you can lift between 15 and 25 times. The increased number of repetitions means you are challenging the slow-twitch muscle fibers for a minute or more. This gets them better at taking in oxygen and at contracting over and over. The weight should be challenging by the time you get to the final reps, and you should work to failure. For endurance workouts, you will lift the weight a little faster than when doing the size or strength routines, and you will not hold the weight in the contracted position. Take about one or two seconds to lift the weight and then immediately lower it, which should take about two seconds. Although the movement is quick, you should always feel as though you are in control of it—don't use momentum to assist you in performing it. (An example of using momentum on a bench press is bouncing the bar off your chest in order to help you lift the weight.) You might need to modify the exercise when it starts getting difficult. For example, when doing a push-up, you can start on your toes, and then when you get tired and start losing your form you can put your knees on the floor and continue.

Power

Perhaps your goal is to increase power. Think of power as the capacity to produce force, like when you are riding up a steep hill while cycling. Everyone ought to do a power workout once in a while. Power exercises are often plyometric movements like lunges and squat jumps, in which you change direction quickly.

Being able to produce force quickly is great if you want to be better at a sport—for example, it means you can hit a golf ball more strongly. Power affects much more than just sports performance, however. It also dictates how quickly you can produce or create a movement or change the direction of your body. In the simplest sense, power is what allows you to get up off a chair quickly and to walk up the stairs without assistance. Let's look at plyometric push-ups, as an example. Doing plyometric push-ups gets your shoulders and arms better at controlling your body's response to the forces on it during the exercise. You can then call on this control for other things you might want to do during the day, such as tossing your kid up in the air for fun.

If developing greater power is a main goal for you, you'll be glad to know that the appropriate workouts will fit easily into your allotted morning time slot. Power workouts are relatively brief, since you can't do many repetitions when you are using so much energy for each one. When doing these workouts, work up to about 10 repetitions of each exercise, although this will be challenging. For example, when you start doing the squat jumps, you will probably find it difficult to do more than two in a row, especially if your squat is deep enough to get your thighs parallel to the floor. Take a second or two after each repetition so that you feel ready for the next one. If you can do 10 reps this way without much difficulty, try to do the movement deeper and try to do the squats consecutively, without any rest at all. Ten reps is also my recommendation for the strength workouts, but the demands of the two types of exercise are quite different. In contrast to the controlled movements of strength training, exercises for power require explosive action. Your heart rate will immediately go up during a power set, and getting to 10 reps will make you feel much more tired overall than 10 reps of a strength workout. Since these movements use more energy, this book has only 20- and 30-minute routines designed exclusively for power. The 45- and 60-minute power workouts are rounded out with core stability exercises and cardio intervals.

General Health and Fitness

This book also offers workouts that are perfect for you if your goal is to enhance your general state of health and fitness. What does that mean? In reading the previous descriptions of strength, size, endurance, and power, did you find yourself thinking that none of that is really what's important to you? Maybe you feel satisfied with the way you look, you usually have enough energy to get through the day, and you just want to maintain that level of fitness as you get older. Perhaps you want to be able to do a set of 10 push-ups or go on a nice bike ride without your legs giving out on you. If your goal is to achieve a higher level of fitness for basic health benefits, not necessarily to get bigger or stronger, then the workouts for general health and fitness in the book will be perfect for you. Working out for general health and fitness means your joints will stay healthy, and you'll be fit enough to play that tennis game on the weekend. These workouts are well rounded, using a variety of equipment so that you don't get bored. The major thing that sets these routines apart from the others is that they don't have you challenge yourself with as much weight as you would for more specific fitness-oriented goals. What better way to start your day than with a workout for general health? Your workouts will increase your bone density, regulate your blood sugar levels, improve your energy level and metabolism, and keep your joints healthy—all before you get to work! You will feel confident all day knowing that you've done something so positive for yourself in the morning.

When you do the routines for general health and fitness, pick a weight that you can comfortably lift between 8 and 12 times. The resistance should be heavy enough for your muscles to be fatigued by the 12th repetition. Fatigue is not the same as failure; it doesn't mean that you are unable to continue, but simply that you feel a little challenged. Try to do a workout for general health and fitness at least two times each week.

Integrated Strength Training

No matter what your main goal is for your strength training program, all workouts have one thing in common: the need for integrated training. The term *integrated strength training* implies that there are more components to your exercise program than just the weight you lift. Integrated strength training means you address other elements of fitness, such as joint stability and balance, that are just as important as the ability to lift weights. Being fit means, among other things, that you can stand on one leg without losing your balance. It also means you can lie on a stability ball without falling off, because your core muscles are strong and your neuromuscular system can keep your body still on an unstable object. These aspects of fitness are important to your daily life. Having a strong core, for example, is important in keeping your low back healthy and performing exercises safely. This section explains the benefits of the elements of integrated training. The workouts in this book include these components.

The following components are important for a well-balanced, or integrated, strength training program:

• **Develop core integrity.** Core integrity means being aware of your core, or midsection. It also means being able to recruit, or use, these muscles when you need more support, as in weightlifting. Our sedentary lifestyle has made it less and less important to have a strong core, because most people no longer do much of the manual labor in which the body really needs to work as a unit to lift and move things. But being aware of your core muscles and deliberately engaging them when you lift weights are important for getting stronger and bigger. When your core is strong, you can lift more weight with your arms and legs.

The workouts in this book include exercises that target your core muscles. Exercises in which you use your body weight against gravity generally work your core as well—push-ups, for example, challenge your core muscles in addition to your chest and arms. There are also exercises that specifically challenge your ability to keep your core muscles engaged and add difficulty by having you move your arms or your legs, like the toe-tap exercises. The core exercises are listed and explained in chapter 11.

- **Work along various planes of motion.** The muscles of your body produce movement by pulling on your bones. Your body is capable of moving in various directions. Although traditional exercises have you move in straight lines (think of a bicep curl or leg extension), that is not how the muscles attach to your bones. If you follow the line of muscle fibers from where they attach to two bones, you will see that they run along a diagonal line, not a straight line. Think of a plane as a sheet of glass that divides your body into two halves. The sagittal plane divides your body into two sides, left and right. When you move along this plane, you are moving forward and backward. A forward lunge is an example of moving along the sagittal plane. The frontal plane divides your body into two sides, front and back. When you move along this plane, you are moving to either side. A lateral lunge is an example of this. The horizontal plane divides your body into two parts, above and below, or a top and bottom half. Movement along this plane is rotation. A standing rotation exercise and a golf swing are examples of moving along the horizontal plane. Your muscles constantly lengthen and shorten in more than one plane at once. This is evident in watching a baseball pitcher get ready to pitch. He coils his body, "winding" it up to store energy. He then unwinds, allowing the entire chain of the body to release the energy and the ball at the end of the chain.

  If you always lift weights in exactly the same way, moving along the same angle and creating the same pattern, that is what your body gets used to. Your joints become good at handling that precise stress, but not the stress of other, different positions. It's frustrating to pull a muscle just because you've tried to do something different, whether during a leisure activity or an everyday task such as putting a load of laundry up on a shelf and turning around to speak to someone at the same time. Changing the angles slightly in your workouts improves your body's ability to handle those changes of position without mishap.

- **Add rotation.** Similarly to working along various planes of movement, it is a good idea to incorporate rotation into your exercises. If you look at the way muscles attach to bones, you will find that the muscle fibers don't actually run in a straight line. All muscles rotate to some degree as part of their actions. For example, the fibers of pectoralis major, or your chest muscle, run along the front of your body and attach to the front, not the inside, of your arm. Because of this, when the pecs contract they rotate the arm internally. When an exercise involves rotation, it often means you can contract the targeted muscles more effectively. Adding rotation to an exercise is easy. When doing a standing cable row and pulling with your right arm, for example, you can rotate your upper body a little to the right as you do the pulling movement. Other exercises in this book that incorporate rotation are the standing rotation with cable or tubing, rotation lunge with dumbbells, and the seated rotation with dumbbell.

- **Work against gravity.** You can do this from a standing, sitting, or lying position. An important benefit of doing exercises that make you stand up or move against gravity is that you have to hold up and move your body yourself, instead of sitting on a machine to do the exercise and letting it support your body. This means you are working your body in accordance with the way it was designed—to be used in movement against the ground! When you do an exercise in which you have to control your entire body in relation to the ground and gravity, the thousands of nerve endings on the soles of your feet start a chain reaction all the way up your body to produce and control every movement you make. In our sedentary society, it is easy to live without fully developing this exquisite connection between the brain and the body. Sometimes, of course, sitting on a machine to do an exercise is a valid choice. The machine can help you stabilize yourself, allowing you to lift additional weight. However, I do encourage you to vary your routines, and at least sometimes do the exercises where you need to move your body against the ground.

Moving on the ground against gravity is also important in increasing bone density. The prevalence of osteoporosis makes this an important part of any fitness program. When you lift weight in any manner, you are encouraging the body to lay down bone materials, since the action of muscles pulling against the bones stimulates this process. We have also learned that the impact from jumping helps increase bone density—jump lunges and squats are great choices for this.

- **Move arms and legs at the same time.** Using exercises that challenge your upper and lower body at the same time increases the demand on your neuromuscular system, making your nervous system work with your muscles to coordinate the movement. This is in keeping with a holistic definition of fitness. It will improve your coordination and enable you not only to look fit but also to be more fit in all aspects of your physical life, whatever challenges you take on. I remember once seeing a bodybuilder colleague from the health club try to play volleyball. He was very developed muscularly, but he couldn't move his arms and legs at the same time! In terms of the efficiency of your morning workouts, you will get more done in less time if you incorporate some of these exercises, such as the standing single-arm chest press and lunge with cable, or the standing lateral lunge with single-arm horizontal row and tubing that are in this book.

- **Use various types of equipment.** Use your body, machines, cables, free weights, and tools like stability balls, tubing, and medicine balls. Exercise is all about stimulating your body to change. If you do the same routines over and over again, your muscles get familiar with the movement, and each time you work out they will need to work a little less hard. By using different equipment, you force your muscles to constantly adjust and work hard. This is especially valuable in the morning, when you want to be efficient with your time and do the most effective workout possible.

- **Challenge your balance.** Standing on one leg while you do an upper-body exercise makes your body's nervous system communicate better with your muscles, since you must constantly adjust your position. Balance is not a conscious act, but a reactive one. You have sensory organs throughout your body that are responsible for sending messages concerning your position in space; what they do is called *proprioception*. You will feel these slight adjustments around your ankle as you try to stand on one leg. Tweaking your morning programs to incorporate this kind of challenge can improve your balance and coordination, help you be more stable in case you want to try some unfamiliar leisure or sport activities, and generally make you work a little harder without having to commit more time to your morning routines.

Workout Intensity

The weight that you lift for a certain number of repetitions, the type of equipment you are using, and any other variables you are manipulating, such as balance, all come together to give you a sense of how "hard" a given exercise or an entire workout is. This is the question of intensity, but not in the traditional sense of the word.

In exercise, the word *intensity* has traditionally referred to the resistance, or weight, that you are lifting—the heavier the weight, the more intense the exercise. This terminology made sense when strength training programs were based on the bodybuilding routines designed to get people bigger and nothing else. As you know from the discussion of integrated training earlier in this chapter, there are many ways to make workouts easier or harder that go beyond just lifting heavier or lighter weights, and the workouts in this book reflect that. With an integrated approach to strength training, intensity takes on a whole new meaning. It has to do with how difficult you feel something is overall, not just the heaviness of the weight you are lifting. When you incorporate components like balance, moving along different angles, and using a stability ball, for example, what you experience as difficult or challenging is a very personal thing. It is purely subjective—the same exercise can feel different to different people, and the same exercise can feel different to the same person at different times depending on the circumstances of a particular workout. You might find it very challenging to use a stability ball instead of a bench for the single-arm rows, while someone else might not perceive that to be difficult. You might find it easy to incorporate a balance challenge into your routine one day but find it harder the next time you try it—perhaps because you didn't sleep well the night before and are having trouble focusing, or because you twisted your ankle during your run the previous day.

There are a couple of ways you can measure intensity. One tool to help you articulate the difficulty of something is the rating of perceived exertion, or RPE. The RPE is a series of numbers along which you rate how hard an exercise or routine feels. I suggest using a scale of 1 to 10. A 1 means that the activity you are doing is not challenging at all, like sitting on the couch watching TV. A 10 means that the activity is as hard as it could possibly be for you at this moment. The results of this type of self-rated scale will be very specific to you, which is right in keeping with the spirit of these morning workouts. For example, if you are doing a 30-minute endurance workout, you should be able to do between 15 and 25 repetitions of each exercise. A weightlifting exercise would be considered hard if you got to 22 reps and absolutely could not lift the weight another time.

On a scale of 1 to 10, that would equal a rating of 9 or 10. If you underestimated the weight and stopped at 25 reps even though you could have gotten to 40, that would probably score as 5 out of 10, meaning it was a little challenging but not that difficult. Remember that RPE can refer both to a given individual exercise and to an entire routine. If you do a challenging routine that rates 8 or 9 on the RPE scale, but it includes an abdominal exercise that only rates a 4 or 5, that's your indication that you need to make that particular exercise more challenging next time. Regardless of the weight you lift, you might notice that a workout with machines is easier than a similar workout using a stability ball, and so you would rate the former lower on the RPE scale.

Another way to take measure of how hard you are working is to think of the entire workout as being low, moderate, or high intensity. Weight, balance, stability, and all the other variables that have been discussed can affect whether you find a workout more or less intense. The purpose of the following explanations is to help you become aware of how hard you are working and understand how to change the perceived intensity of your workout for maximal efficiency.

Low-Intensity Workouts

Think of the words *low intensity* (also known as *light*) in the sense of easy, or not too challenging. Now, what is easy for you might not be easy for the next person. You might find it easy to use a stability ball, and for someone else this might be extremely difficult or even impossible. Think of a low-intensity workout as one where you are maintaining your fitness level but not actively working to improve it—not really pushing yourself. If your main goal is to develop endurance, your strength training program will require you to lift a weight between 15 and 25 repetitions. In a low-intensity workout, you might do 15 reps, but that's it. That would translate to an RPE of about 4 or 5 out of 10. You can also think of a light workout as one in which you exercise without challenging yourself in any areas that are particularly difficult for you. For example, if you find it difficult to use a stability ball instead of a bench, then you would just stick to using the bench in a light workout. If you find it difficult to do cardio intervals in your workout, then you'd leave them out of a light workout.

Low-intensity workouts are great for several reasons. If you just don't feel like exercising on a given morning, you can promise yourself that you will at least go through the motions and get *some* benefit. You might find that once you get started, you feel motivated to turn it into a more challenging routine! If you are feeling distracted, you can go through an easy routine to clear your mind and help you prepare for the rest of your day. If you are in an unfamiliar gym, you can do an easy workout that doesn't involve much equipment so you don't have to look around for things like tubing or stability balls. In summary, think of a workout of low intensity as one where your repetitions are at the lower end of the suggested range and you don't incorporate any variables that would be especially challenging.

Moderate-Intensity Workouts

Think of moderate-intensity workouts as the in-between kind. When you do one, you are definitely challenging yourself but not working to failure. You stay in the middle range of the recommended repetitions. You might do the same exercises as in a light workout but use more resistance, do a few more repetitions, or repeat the exercises several times to make the entire workout longer. Maybe you perceive the workout you did this morning as light because you could have done 25 reps of the exercises but only did 15 reps. For the next workout, you might push yourself a little more and do 20 reps of each exercise to make the routine a little more challenging, or of moderate intensity. You could add one of the other variables that you find difficult. For example, if your light workout was done with dumbbells and a bench, you could substitute the stability ball for the bench to challenge your balance and core stability a little more. Or you might pick one of the workouts that has you do cardio intervals on a bike in between the exercises if that is what you perceive as being more challenging. A moderate workout translates to an RPE of about 6 or 7.

High-Intensity Workouts

Your high-intensity workouts are the ones in which you push yourself and challenge yourself in as many capacities as you desire. An intense workout demands focus and attention. In a high-intensity workout, your repetitions are toward the high end of the suggested range. If the suggested range is 15 to 25 reps, you would try to do 25 reps. Each exercise, and the routine as a whole, would rate 9 or 10 on the RPE scale. These workouts are also the ones that incorporate more than one of the variables of integrated training, such as challenging your balance and working along various planes of movement. You might stand on one leg to do your shoulder presses or balance on one leg in between your walking lunges. High-intensity workouts are necessary if you have a very specific goal you need to reach by a certain time. For example, suppose you are a cyclist and you notice that you get very tired during the last few miles of your rides. If you have an important race coming up, you need to work at a high intensity to get ready for that performance. The more driven you are to achieve your fitness goals within a certain period of time, the more intense your workouts need to be.

Tracking Your Workouts

Now that you have all the information you need to plan your workouts, you should think about how you will keep a record of your program. Keeping a workout log is valuable for a number of reasons. Putting what you do in writing is a great way to make sure you're staying on track to reach your goals. It can help you be more efficient in your morning routines, since you will always know what you did last time—that way you'll grab the exact dumbbell you need, instead of starting with a weight that is too light and not realizing it until you have finished a set. A workout log can also inspire you to keep going by showing you all the progress you've been making over time.

Besides recording your workouts, you also might find it helpful and motivating to keep track of other components of your lifestyle and fitness program, such as nutrition, body weight, and sleep habits, as explained in chapter 1. As with your workouts, when you write this information down it becomes more concrete; you see it right in front of you and refer back to it each morning. This can be a powerful tool to help you stay on track to reach your goals.

Table 5.1 is a sample blank weekly program log where you can record your goals and your progress. You can also use it to log the additional variables just mentioned, such as how you are sleeping. The column marked "Notes" can be used for miscellaneous things you might like to record, such as your stress levels or something particular that happens during the day that might affect your energy or motivation. Table 5.2 is a sample blank individual workout log that you can use to record information about each of your individual workouts, such as which workout you picked, how many sets and repetitions you did, and how much weight you used. Table 5.3 is a weekly program log that is filled in as an example. Table 5.4 is a sample individual workout log that is filled in.

Rest and Overtraining

It is very important to take occasional days off from exercising. Exercise places stress on the body, and the body's response to this stress is what we call results! The sliding filament theory describes how the protein filaments within muscle fibers glide across each other and grab on to each other in order to shorten the muscle fibers. When you impose a demand on your muscles by lifting a weight to the point at which it is virtually impossible to continue, a series of chemical reactions takes place, making those muscle fibers thicker and stronger in order to be able to handle that demand the next time. Stimulating your muscles by lifting weights is only one part of the picture—you also need proper nutrition and plenty of rest to get the results you want.

It can take several days for your muscle fibers to recover from the stimulus and stress of weight training, especially if your workouts are intense. If you do another workout before your muscles have fully recovered, you will not be strong enough to get the most out of the exercise. It also means that the energy your body would normally use to replenish the glycogen stores in your muscles is being diverted to do another workout. How hard you work during the workout can affect how much rest you need before the next one. If you do light or moderate workouts, then working two or even three mornings in a row will not hurt your results. But if you always work to failure and you are doing a lot of sets and reps, then a day between workouts is a necessary component of your program.

Table 5.1 **Weekly Program Log**

Week of _____

Goal: _____

Progress made toward goal: _____

Day/date	Wake-up/ sleep time	Energy: waking/noon/ 3 p.m./8 p.m.	Eating	Notes
Sunday				
Monday				
Tuesday				
Wednesday				
Thursday				
Friday				
Saturday				

From *Morning Strength Workouts* by Annette Lang, 2007, Champaign, IL: Human Kinetics.

Table 5.2 **Individual Workout Log**

Date of workout: _____

Type/length of workout: _____

Exercise	Weight/reps	Notes

From *Morning Strength Workouts* by Annette Lang, 2007, Champaign, IL: Human Kinetics.

Table 5.3 Sample Completed Weekly Program Log

Week of _5/14–5/20_

Goal: _Complete more reps with strength workouts. Finish bike rides feeling strong._

Progress made toward goal: _I am feeling better on the bike; endurance workouts are helping!_

Day/date	Wake-up/ sleep time	Energy: waking/noon/ 3 p.m./8 p.m.	Eating	Notes
Sunday 5/14	9/11	Very high/very high/high/high	Cereal at 9:30; nuts and banana on bike ride; veggie burger, fries, salad at 5 p.m.; 2 beers	40-mile bike ride; felt great!
Monday 5/15	7/12	High/high/low/ high	Yogurt, banana at 7:30; chocolate cake at 3 p.m.; huge salad with grilled salmon at 7 p.m.; not enough water	Shouldn't have skipped lunch— stop skipping lunch!
Tuesday 5/16	6:30/11	Low/moderate/ high/high	Yogurt and banana before wkt., cereal after; soup and half sandwich at noon; grapes and orange in the afternoon; pasta and veggies at 8 p.m.; 1 glass wine	Felt better after workout.
Wednesday 5/17	7/10:30	High/high/high/ low	Muffin at 7; apple; salad with tuna on top at 1 p.m.; watermelon; Chinese food at 8 p.m.	Bike ride after work.
Thursday 5/18	6:30/12	Very high/ moderate/low/ very high	Cereal and yogurt after wkt.; banana; grilled veggies and shrimp at noon; huge salad with tofu at 7 p.m.; several beers at party	Workout felt high intensity—am tired.
Friday 5/19	7:15/1	Low/low/low/ high	2 doughnuts at work; 2 slices pizza; huge salad and veggies	Had a late night, but had fun!
Saturday 5/20	8/11	Very high/high/ high/high	Brunch; egg-white omelet with veggies, Bloody Mary; sushi, salad in evening	Nice easy bike ride; took a nap— felt great!

Table 5.4   **Sample Completed Individual Workout Log**

Date of workout: *5/16*

Type/length of workout: *30-minute workout for endurance; 1 set of each; 15–25 reps.*

Warm-up/stretches/SMR/corrective exercises: *core warm-up; hip flexor stretch.*

Exercise	Weight/reps	Notes
Squat w/dumbbells	20/20	2 more than last time!
Walking lunge w/rotation and med ball	4 lb ball, 21 reps	
Lat roll-out on stability ball	15	Felt hard today; RPE=9
Prone hold on stability ball	5 circles	
Push-up	17, 6 more on knees	Got to get to 20! Maybe do these more often at home?
Standing single-arm chest press w/tubing	19 reps	
Standing single-arm shoulder press w/tubing	26 reps	Increase resistance next time.
Standing lateral lunge w/single-arm hor. row and tubing	21 reps	
Toe tap	1 min	Core is definitely getting stronger; these felt great.
Opposite arm/leg reach	23	
Prone hold on hands	30 sec	
Bridge w/lower body on stability ball	22	
Back extension	20	
Walking lunge w/ dumbbells	12/20	Balance felt a little off; tired?
Straight-arm pull-down w/cable	4 plates/20	

Overtraining is what happens when you exercise too often, with insufficient rest between workouts. It means that instead of benefiting from your workouts, you are actually wearing your body down. You should be aware of several factors to determine whether you are overtraining. One major question is whether you are getting stronger, bigger, leaner (or closer to whatever goal you have set). Basically, are you getting the results that you want? If your body is constantly tired because you are doing high-intensity strength workouts every morning and not resting enough, it cannot catch up in order to actually improve in whatever area is important to you. Another way to judge whether you are overtraining is to pay attention to your resting heart rate. Taking your pulse for one full minute in the morning when you wake up will give you your resting heart rate. To take your pulse, put your index and middle fingers on your neck by your carotid artery, which is located just to either side of the center of your neck. When you can feel your pulse, or heart rate, count it for one full minute. A normal resting heart rate is between 60 and 90 beats per minute. The most important thing is to notice any change in yourself. If your heart rate is higher than it used to be, you might be overtraining. An elevated heart rate means that your body is not catching up—it's getting too little rest between workouts to recover, and it's working harder than it should be. Exercising regularly should gradually slow down your resting heart rate—this is a sign that your heart is getting stronger and therefore no longer needs to contract as many times during the day as it used to. Another possible sign that you are working too hard or not taking enough time off between workouts is that you feel your energy level is down from what you consider normal for you. Exercise should make you feel more energetic, not less!

Becoming aware of your daily habits and workout routine by using the logs in this chapter can help you notice any trouble spots and stay on target to reach your goals. You are putting a lot of mental and physical energy into your morning routines, and with a little attention to these things, you will be successful.

Workouts for Every Schedule

6

20-Minute Programs

Twenty-minute routines are valuable for working out in the morning. For a small time investment, you can get a decent workout that will help you feel energized. Doing a quick workout first thing in the morning also contributes to a positive mindset, encouraging you to stay on track with your other goals, such as eating better or taking a brisk walk at lunchtime. An efficient 20-minute routine is useful if your morning strength training routine is part of a longer workout that might include cardiovascular exercise, Pilates, or yoga. You can also use a 20-minute routine as part of an exercise program that you begin in the morning and complete at the end of your workday. For example, you might do a 20-minute routine in the morning and then go for a run or bike ride after work.

It is also easy to lengthen your 20-minute morning workout. If you get up and find that your morning schedule has changed so that you have some extra time, or if once you get into the workout you just decide to keep going, you can do the workout twice. On the other hand, a 20-minute routine is perfect for the times when you've planned to do a longer workout but wake up late or feeling a little tired. It will get your blood flowing, increase your heart rate, and wake you up for the rest of your day. Sometimes it's good to "go through the motions," even if you don't have the time or energy for a heavy-duty routine. It will help you stay on track to achieve your overall fitness goals. Pick a warm-up from chapter 4 before starting the workout.

20-Minute Workout for Strength

This workout uses more machines than other types of equipment. When your goal is to build strength, you need to lift relatively heavy weights, and machines allow you to do that because they provide support for your body. They also allow you to focus solely on the mechanics of the movement itself, instead of on two or more things at once as in some of the other routines that challenge your balance, for example, at the same time as your strength. This workout is a good choice if you are going to the gym, since you can probably find all the equipment you need there. It is designed to work your lower body first and then your

1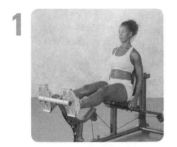

Leg Press
Page 214

2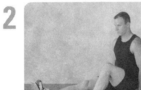

Single-Leg Press
Page 215

3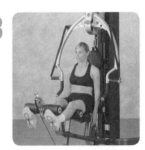

Leg Extension
Page 216

4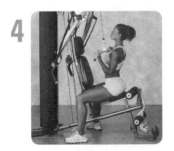

Lat Pull-Down
Page 140

5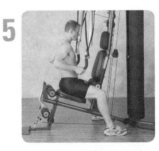

Row on Machine
Page 139

6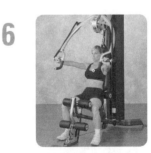

Seated Chest Press
on Machine
Page 156

upper body. This can save you time looking for machines, since most gyms organize their equipment according to muscle groups and areas of the body. The lower-body machines should be in close proximity to each other; when you finish with them you can go to the upper-body machines to complete the routine.

Do this routine one time through. Refer to chapter 5 for recommendations on picking the correct weight for strength workouts. Do 8 to 10 repetitions of each exercise.

7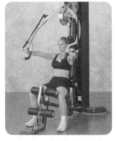

Seated Chest Press on Machine
Note: Repeat the exercise
with one arm at a time.
Page 156

8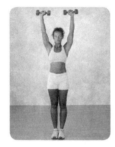

**Standing Shoulder Press
With Dumbbells**
Page 157

9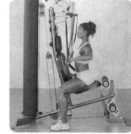

Horizontal Row on Machine
Page 164

10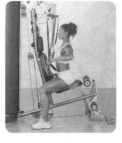

Horizontal Row on Machine
Note: Repeat the exercise
with one arm at a time.
Page 164

11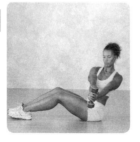

**Seated Rotation With
Dumbbell**
Note: Rotate very slowly.
Page 179

20-Minute Workout for Size

In keeping with the concept of integrated training explained in chapter 5, many of the exercises in this routine make you work on additional elements of fitness besides just lifting weight. The lateral lunge and the standing exercises challenge your core. The biceps curl challenges your balance by having you stand on one leg as you do the exercise. This routine is a good choice if you wake up feeling like you've slept enough and are in good shape to work a little harder and focus on these different variables.

Do this routine one time through. Refer to chapter 5 for guidelines on what weight you should use for routines aimed at increasing muscular size. Do 10 to 15 repetitions of each exercise.

1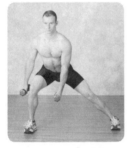

Lateral Lunge With Dumbbells
Page 203

2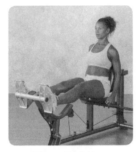

Leg Press
Page 214

3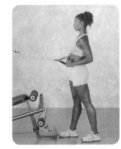

Row With Cable
Note: **Row with cable coming from straight ahead.**
Page 138

4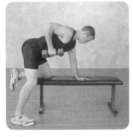

Single-Arm Row With Dumbbell on Bench
Page 134

5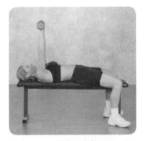

Chest Press With Dumbbells on Bench
Page 151

6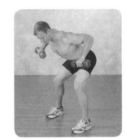

Standing Horizontal Row With Dumbbells
Page 160

7

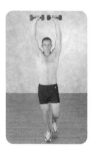

**Single-Leg Standing Biceps
Curl Into Shoulder Press
With Dumbbells
Page 158**

8

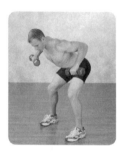

**Standing Horizontal Row
With Dumbbells**
Note: Alternate arms.
Page 160

9

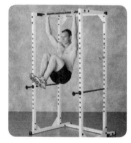

**Hanging Leg Raise
Page 178**

10

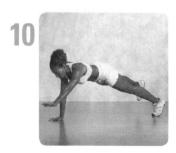

Crab Walk
Note: 10 steps to each side.
Page 189

20-Minute Workout for Endurance

This workout starts with a core challenge and is therefore perfect if you feel like you've been a bit lazy with your core exercises lately, or if you want to give your posture or low back an extra boost. Starting with core exercises helps your whole body wake up, since your core connects your upper and lower body. Your core will continue to be challenged as you do the other exercises. The high number of repetitions in this endurance routine means that you will really feel this workout for the rest of the day—a little "burn" to remind you of what you've accomplished!

Do this workout one time through. Refer to chapter 5 for specifics about picking the right weight for developing endurance. Do 15 to 25 repetitions of each exercise.

1
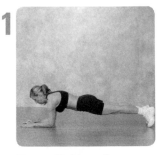

Prone Hold on Forearms
Note: Hold up to 20 seconds.
Page 174

2
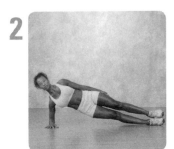

Lateral Hold on Forearm
Note: Hold up to 20 seconds on each side.
Page 176

3
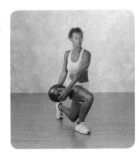

Walking Lunge With Rotation and Medicine Ball
Page 202

4
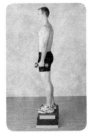

Step-Up With Dumbbells
Page 206

5
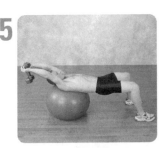

Pull-Over With Dumbbell on Stability Ball
Page 143

6

Horizontal Row With Cable
Note: Alternate arms.
Page 161

7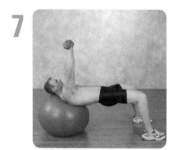

**Chest Press With Dumbbells
on Stability Ball
Page 153**

8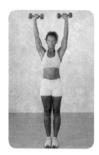

**Standing Shoulder Press
With Dumbbells
Page 157**

9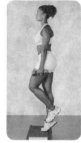

**Single-Leg Heel Raise With
Dumbbell
Page 212**

10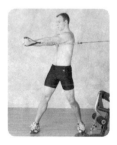

**Standing Rotation With Cable
Page 181**

20-Minute Workout for Power

This workout demands attention and focus, so it is a good choice for a morning when you feel rested and refreshed. It is also a great choice when you want to work out outdoors, as discussed in chapter 2. You can also do this at the gym or at home. If you do it at home and don't have a cable rack or bar to use for the chin-ups, substitute another lat or pulling exercise. Rest for as long as you need to between the exercises; if you don't get through it all in 20 minutes, that's OK.

Do this workout one time through. Refer to chapter 5 for guidelines on how to pick a weight for your power routines. Depending on your goals, do 3 to 10 repetitions of each exercise unless otherwise noted.

1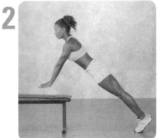

Squat Jump
Page 198

2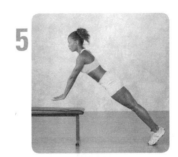

Plyometric Push-Up Against Bench
Page 150

3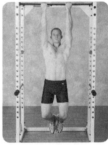

Negative Chin-Up
Note: Lower yourself in 10 seconds.
Page 145

4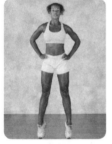

Jump Lunge
Page 205

5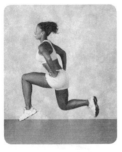

Plyometric Push-Up Against Bench
Page 150

6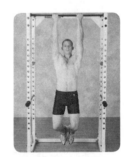

Negative Chin-Up
Note: Lower yourself in 10 seconds.
Page 145

7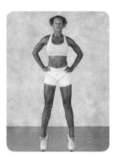

Squat Jump
Page 198

8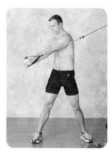

Standing Chop With Cable
Note: 30 seconds on
each side.
Page 190

9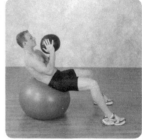

**Crunch on Stability Ball
With Medicine Ball**
Note: One minute.
Page 187

10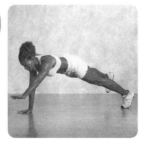

Crab Walk
Note: Move from one side to
the other as space permits
for a total of one minute.
Page 189

20-Minute Workout for General Health and Fitness

This routine balances several different variables—using your weight against gravity, machines, a stability ball, a medicine ball, and a cable—to give you a terrific overall workout. A morning routine for general health and fitness should work your whole body, challenge your neuromuscular system, energize you, and basically just make you feel great, ready to start your day with a smile.

Do this workout one time through. Refer to chapter 5 for guidelines on how to pick the weight for routines for general health and fitness. Do 8 to 12 repetitions of each exercise.

1
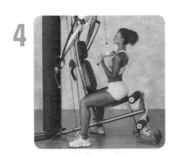
Bridge With Lower Body on Stability Ball
Page 208

2
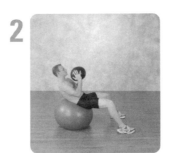
Crunch on Stability Ball With Medicine Ball
Page 187

3
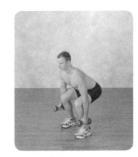
Free-Standing Squat With Dumbbells
Page 194

4
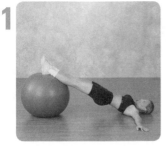
Lat Pull-Down
Page 140

5
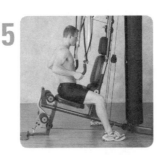
Row on Machine
Page 139

6
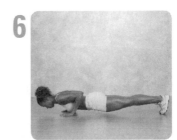
Push-Up
Page 146

7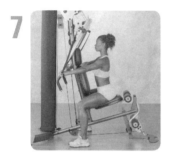

Horizontal Row on Machine
Page 164

8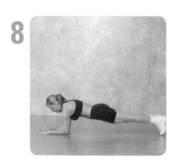

Prone Hold on Forearms
Page 174

9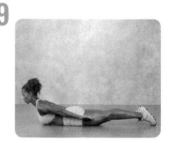

Back Extension
Page 185

10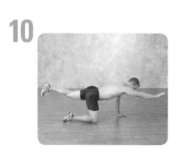

Opposite Arm/Leg Reach
Page 173

7

30-Minute Programs

ΙΙΙΙΙΙΙΙΙΙΙΙΙΙΙΙΙΙΙΙΙΙΙΙΙΙΙΙΙΙΙΙΙΙΙΙΙΙΙΙΙΙΙΙΙΙΙΙΙΙΙΙΙΙΙΙΙΙΙΙΙΙΙΙΙΙΙΙΙΙΙΙΙΙΙΙΙΙΙΙΙΙΙΙΙΙΙΙΙΙΙΙΙΙΙΙΙΙΙΙΙΙΙΙΙΙΙΙΙΙΙΙΙΙΙΙΙΙΙ

A 30-minute workout obviously gives you 10 minutes more than a 20-minute workout, extra time that you can use to fit in one or two things you don't have time for in the shorter routine. For example, you can push yourself a little harder, getting in some additional repetitions. If you have 10 extra minutes in the morning, you can also stick with one of the 20-minute routines and use the extra time to do a longer warm-up if you feel you need it or a few extra minutes of stretching.

Doing 30-minute routines in the morning instead of 20-minute ones can help you be more efficient in your overall fitness program. For example, if you do two 30-minute routines each week instead of three 20-minute routines, you'll spend the same total amount of time strength training, but you will also have an extra morning every week that you can use to do another type of activity such as a cardiovascular workout, yoga, or Pilates. If your program goals are more related to muscle size and endurance, however, a 30-minute workout means that your muscles will get a greater volume of training per session, which simply means that they will spend more time under tension, leading to potentially better results in terms of muscular size, muscular endurance, and the like. So you can use these different routines to plan a comprehensive program tailored to your goals and preferences.

30-Minute Workout for Strength

For this workout, do two sets of each exercise, resting 30 seconds between sets. Doing the same exercise twice in a row makes the second set especially challenging for the targeted muscle group. This type of routine is nice in the morning since you don't have to do many different exercises—it's a good choice for days when you don't feel like concentrating on what comes next, because you're still feeling a little dreamy or your mind is preoccupied with the upcoming workday.

Refer to chapter 5 for specifics on how much weight you should use for your strength workout. Do 8 to 10 repetitions of each exercise for each set.

1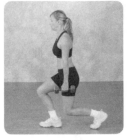

**Reverse Lunge With
Dumbbells
Page 200**

2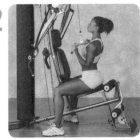

**Lat Pull-Down
Page 140**

3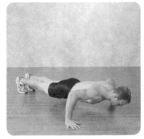

**Walking Push-Up
Page 148**

4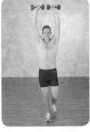

**Single-Leg Standing Biceps
Curl Into Shoulder Press
With Dumbbells
Page 158**

5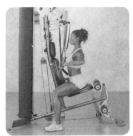

**Horizontal Row on Machine
Page 164**

6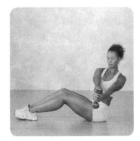

**Seated Rotation With
Dumbbell
Page 179**

7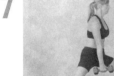
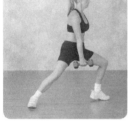

**Rotation Lunge With
Dumbbells
Page 204**

8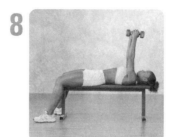

**Pull-Over With Dumbbell
on Bench
Page 142**

9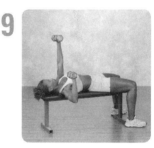

**Alternating Chest Press With
Dumbbells on Bench
Page 152**

10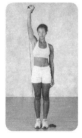

**Standing Single-Arm
Shoulder Press With Tubing
Page 159**

11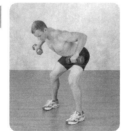

**Standing Horizontal Row
With Dumbbells
Page 160**

12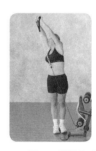

**Reverse Chop With Cable
Page 172**

30-Minute Workout for Size

This is perfect for mornings when you have gotten enough sleep, feel good, and are ready to move quickly from exercise to exercise. Challenging a different area of your body for each new exercise keeps your blood flowing and your heart rate elevated throughout the routine.

Do the entire workout one time through. Refer to chapter 5 for guidelines on how much weight to use for your routines for size. Do 10 to 15 repetitions of each exercise.

1
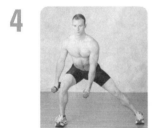
Supine Rotation
Note: Keep legs relatively straight.
Page 184

2
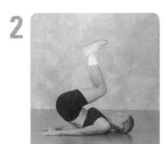
Reverse Crunch
Page 183

3
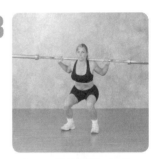
Squat With Barbell
Page 195

4
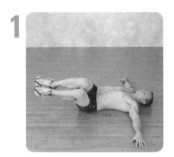
Lateral Lunge With Dumbbells
Note: Alternate sides.
Page 203

5
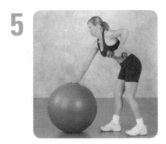
Single-Arm Row With Dumbbell on Stability Ball
Page 135

6
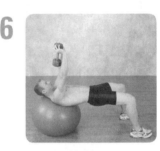
Pull-Over With Dumbbell on Stability Ball
Page 143

7
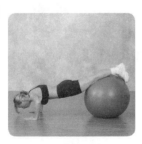
Push-Up With Legs on Stability Ball
Page 149

8
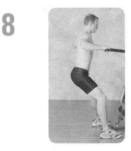
Horizontal Row With Cable
Note: Alternate arms.
Page 161

9
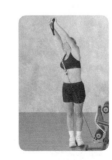
Reverse Chop With Cable
Page 172

10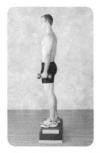

Step-Up With Dumbbells
Page 206

11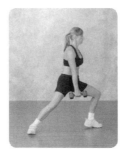

Rotation Lunge
Note: Do all repetitions to the
right side first, then the left side.
Page 204

12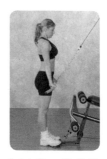

Straight-Arm Pull-Down
With Cable
Page 141

13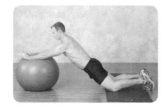

Lat Roll-Out on Stability Ball
Page 144

14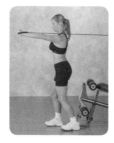

Standing Single-Arm Chest
Press With Tubing
Page 154

15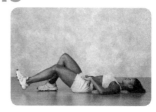

Toe Tap With Longer Leg
Page 170

30-Minute Workout for Endurance

Although this workout does not use machines, it does use a variety of pieces of equipment, so choose this routine when you feel awake and ready for challenges to your core integrity and balance along with many repetitions.

Do this entire workout once. Refer to chapter 5 for suggestions on choosing the weight to lift for endurance exercises. Unless otherwise noted, do 15 to 25 repetitions of each exercise.

1
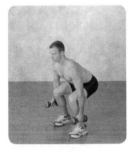

Free-Standing Squat With Dumbbells
Page 194

2
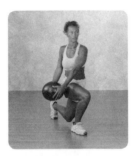

Walking Lunge With Rotation and Medicine Ball
Page 202

3
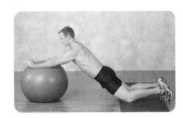

Lat Roll-Out on Stability Ball
Page 144

4
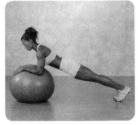

Prone Hold on Stability Ball
Note: 5 circles to each side.
Page 188

5
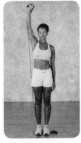

Push-Up
Page 146

6
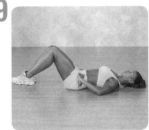

Standing Single-Arm Chest Press With Tubing
Page 154

7

Standing Single-Arm Shoulder Press With Tubing
Page 159

8

Standing Lateral Lunge With Single-Arm Horizontal Row and Tubing
Page 162

9
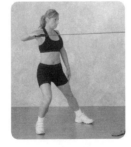

Toe Tap
Note: Up to 1 minute.
Page 169

10
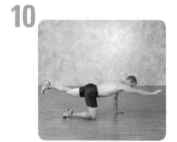

Opposite Arm/Leg Reach
Page 173

11
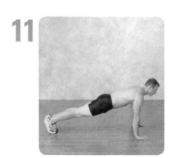

Prone Hold on Hands
Page 175

12
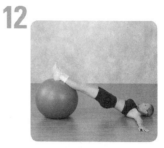

Bridge With Lower Body on
Stability Ball
Page 208

13
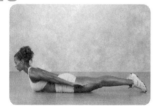

Back Extension
Page 185

14
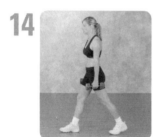

Walking Lunge With
Dumbbells
Page 201

15
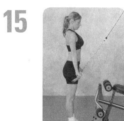

Straight-Arm Pull-Down With
Cable
Page 141

16
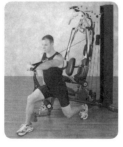

Standing Single-Arm Chest
Press and Lunge With Cable
Page 155

17
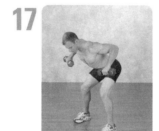

Standing Horizontal Row With
Dumbbells
Note: Alternate arms.
Page 160

18
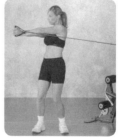

Standing Rotation With
Tubing
Page 180

30-Minute Workout for Power

Some of the exercises in this routine have you focus on deceleration. This means you will emphasize the slowing down of the movement, which requires your muscles and joints to control the position of your body in space. If you are in a gym, especially in the morning when the gym might be crowded or when you might be a little less coordinated, be very careful when you do the medicine ball lifts. The medicine ball needs to be light enough

1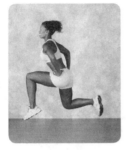

Jump Lunge
Note: Alternate leg position
after each repetition.
Page 205

2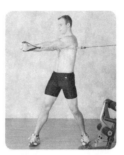

Standing Rotation With Cable
Note: Focus on slowing down
the movement.
Page 181

3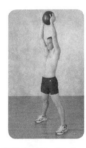

Lat Roll-Out on Stability Ball
Note: Focus on slowing down
the movement.
Page 144

4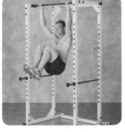

Hanging Leg Raise
Note: Focus on legs
lowering.
Page 178

5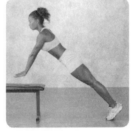

**Plyometric Push-Up Against
Bench**
Page 150

6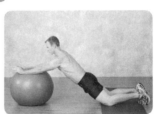

Squat With Medicine Ball Lift
Note: Squat slowly, and lift
the ball overhead quickly.
See figure 4.10 on page 58

7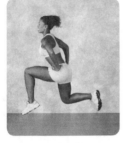

Jump Lunge
Note: Alternate leg position
after each repetition.
Page 205

8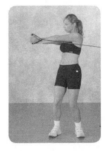

Standing Rotation With Tubing
Note: Focus on slowing
down the movement.
Page 180

9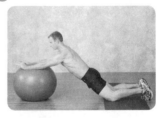

Lat Roll-Out on Stability Ball
Note: Focus on slowing
down the movement.
Page 144

for you to have total confidence in your ability to hold on to it, and you should make sure you are ready and focused before you start the exercise. Some other exercises here focus on your core, which will provide a needed break between the jumping exercises!

Do this workout one time through. See the recommendations in chapter 5 on choosing the weight to use for power exercises. Do 3 to 10 repetitions of each exercise.

10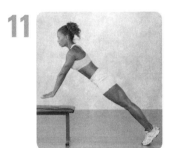

Hanging Leg Raise
Note: Focus on legs lowering.
Page 178

11

Plyometric Push-Up Against Bench
Page 150

12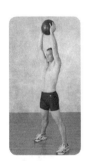

Squat With Medicine Ball Lift
Note: Squat slowly, and lift the ball overhead quickly.
See figure 4.10 on page 58

13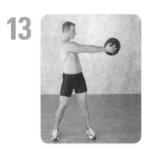

Standing Rotation With Medicine Ball
See figure 4.12 on page 59

30-Minute Workout for General Health and Fitness

This is a nice routine in the morning if you want to alternate a few lower-body exercises with a few upper-body ones. It does not demand too much from any one area of the body at a time.

Do this workout one time through. Refer to chapter 5 for guidelines on choosing weight for routines for general health and fitness. Do 8 to 12 repetitions of each exercise.

1
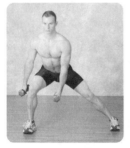
Lateral Lunge With Dumbbells
Page 203

2
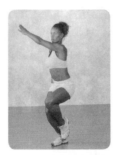
Single-Leg Squat With Opposite-Arm Reach
Page 197

3
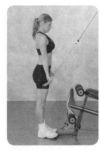
Straight-Arm Pull-Down With Cable
Page 141

4
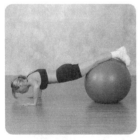
Push-Up With Legs on Stability Ball
Page 149

5
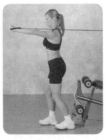
Standing Single-Arm Chest Press With Tubing
Page 154

6
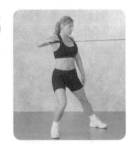
Standing Lateral Lunge With Single-Arm Horizontal Row and Tubing
Page 162

7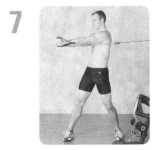

Standing Rotation With Cable
Page 181

8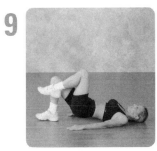

Squat With Medicine Ball Lift
See figure 4.10 on page 58

9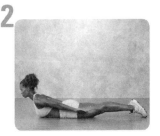

Single-Leg Bridge on Floor
Page 210

10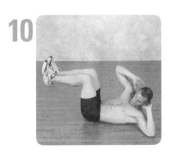

Oblique Crunch
Page 182

11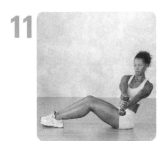

Seated Rotation With Dumbbell
Page 179

12

Back Extension
Page 185

8

45-Minute Programs

||||||||||||||||||||||||||||||||||||||||||||||||||||||||||||||||||||||||||||||||||||||||||||||||||||||||||||||||||||||||||

With 45-minute routines, you have more opportunity to make your workout demanding than with the shorter routines. You can do more exercises, or you can incorporate different challenges into the routine, such as active rest intervals (a core exercise after every set) or cardiovascular intervals (jumping rope for one minute after every set). The latter are a great way to get some cardio exercise into your morning routine, and they're perfect when you want to burn a few extra calories in preparation for an event that evening where you anticipate eating more calories than you normally would. They also get your heart pumping and make you feel ready to go for the day!

45-Minute Workout for Strength

In this workout you will do one set of an exercise, then do a core exercise for 30 seconds (or as long as you can!) as an active rest, and then do another exercise for the same muscle group. You will therefore fatigue the same muscle group over two or more sets. You will do all the lower-body exercises first, fatiguing those muscles before moving to the upper-body exercises. This routine is a great choice in the morning if you want to work a little harder than usual on your core and you have the time to do it. Many people promise themselves

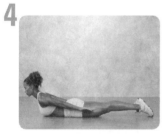

1 Leg Press
Page 214

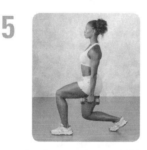

2 Seated Rotation With
Dumbbell
Note: 30 seconds.
Page 179

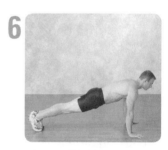

3 Leg Extension
Page 216

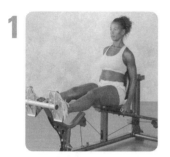

4 Back Extension
Note: 6 repetitions, holding
for 5 seconds each rep.
Page 185

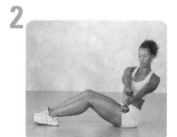

5 Stationary Lunge With
Dumbbells
Page 199

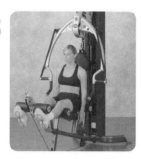

6 Prone Hold on Hands
Note: 30 seconds.
Page 175

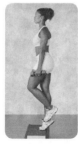

7 Single-Leg Heel Raise
With Dumbbell
Page 212

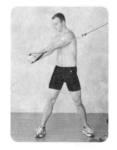

8 Standing Chop With Cable
Note: 30 seconds.
Page 190

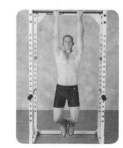

9 Chin-Up or Negative Chin-Up
Page 145

108

that they'll do extra abdominal exercises while watching television at night but don't actually do it when the time comes. Pick this routine if you want to get that core training in first thing so you can feel good about it the rest of the day.

Do this routine one time through. Chapter 5 gives you recommendations for choosing the right weight for strength routines. Do 8 to 10 repetitions of each exercise unless otherwise noted.

10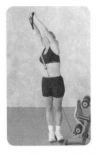

Reverse Chop With Cable
Note: 30 seconds.
Page 172

11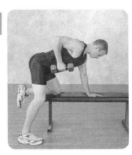

Single-Arm Row With Dumbbell on Bench
Page 134

12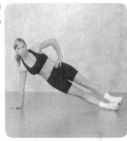

Lateral Hold With Straight Arm
Note: Hold as long as you can or up to 30 seconds on each side.
Page 177

13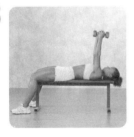

Pull-Over With Dumbbell on Bench
Page 142

14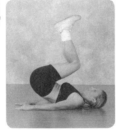

Reverse Crunch
Note: 30 seconds.
Page 183

15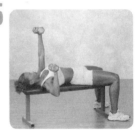

Alternating Chest Press With Dumbbells on Bench
Page 152

16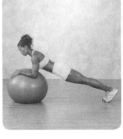

Prone Hold on Stability Ball
Note: 30 seconds.
Page 188

17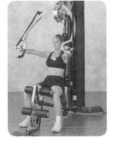

Seated Chest Press on Machine
Page 156

18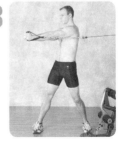

Standing Rotation With Cable
Note: 30 seconds each side.
Page 181

(continued)

19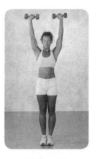

**Standing Shoulder Press
With Dumbbells
Page 157**

20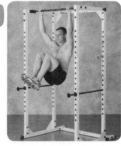

**Hanging Leg Raise
Note: 30 seconds.
Page 178**

21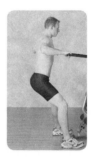

**Horizontal Row With Cable
Page 161**

This routine is a full-body workout and includes at least two exercises for each muscle group. Do the entire routine twice through. See chapter 5 for recommendations on choosing weight for developing muscle size. Do 10 to 15 repetitions of each exercise.

1

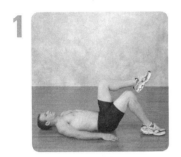

Toe Tap With Both Feet Up
Page 171

2

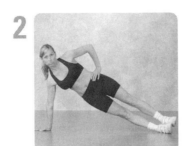

Lateral Hold With
Straight Arm
Page 177

3

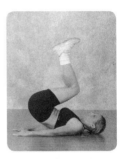

Reverse Crunch
Page 183

4

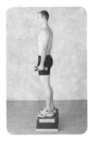

Step-Up With Dumbbells
Page 206

5

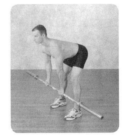

Deadlift With Barbell
Page 207

6

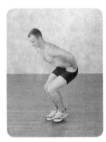

Single-Leg Squat
Page 196

7

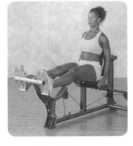

Leg Press
Page 214

8

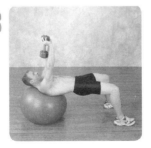

Pull-Over With Dumbbell
on Stability Ball
Page 143

9

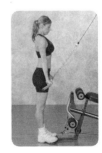

Straight-Arm Pull-Down
With Cable
Page 141

(continued)

10
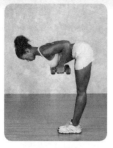

**Unsupported Row With
Dumbbells
Page 136**

11
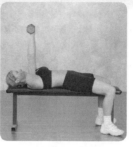

**Chest Press With
Dumbbells on Bench
Page 151**

12
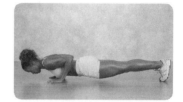

**Push-up
Page 146**

13
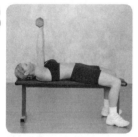

**Chest Press With
Dumbbells on Bench
Note: Alternate arms.
Page 151**

14
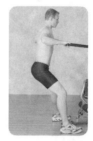

**Horizontal Row With Cable
Page 161**

15
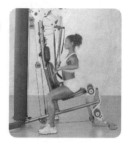

**Horizontal Row
on Machine
Page 164**

16
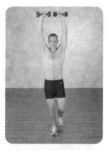

**Single-Leg Standing Biceps
Curl Into Shoulder Press
With Dumbbells
Page 158**

17
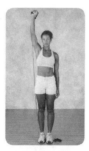

**Standing Single-Arm
Shoulder Press With Tubing
Page 159**

18
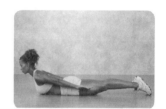

**Back Extension
Page 185**

19
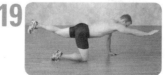

**Opposite Arm/Leg Reach
Page 173**

This is a challenging routine, so catch your breath in between the exercises if you need to! This endurance workout includes cardio intervals. Combining cardiovascular work with your strength training is a great way to make your morning routines efficient. An interval simply means a movement or exercise done for a specific period of time; it traditionally refers to cardiovascular exercise. You can substitute another cardio exercise if the one mentioned is not available. For the jump-rope exercises, if you mess up, just start again and keep going until you get the allotted amount of actual jumping time.

Do this entire routine three times. Refer to chapter 5 for how much weight to lift in endurance routines. Do 15 to 25 repetitions of each exercise unless otherwise noted.

1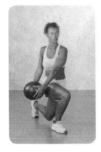

Walking Lunge With Rotation and Medicine Ball
Page 202
Cardio Interval: Jump rope for 1 minute

2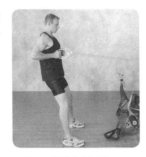

Row With Tubing
Note: Alternate arms.
Page 137
Cardio Interval: Stationary bicycle or treadmill, 3 minutes

3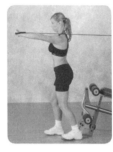

Standing Single-Arm Chest Press With Tubing
Page 154
Cardio Interval: Jump rope for 1 minute

4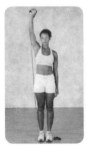

Standing Single-Arm Shoulder Press With Tubing
Page 159
Cardio Interval: Stationary bicycle or treadmill, 3 minutes

5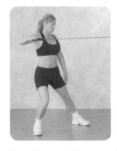

Standing Lateral Lunge With Single-Arm Horizontal Row and Tubing
Page 162
Cardio Interval: Jump rope for 1 minute

6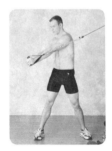

Standing Chop With Cable
Page 190

45-Minute Workout for Power

Since by definition you cannot do many repetitions when you are working really hard, this power routine incorporates some high-intensity cardio intervals in between the exercises, as well as a series of body-weight and core exercises at the end of the workout. Take as much time as you need between exercises and between circuits. Remember, the time that you take to catch your breath gives you a chance to recover, enabling you to work hard again.

Cardio Interval: This explanation uses a stationary bicycle as an example, but you can use another piece of cardio equipment, such as an elliptical machine or a treadmill. The basic principles are the same no matter which piece of equipment you use. For these intervals, pick a level of resistance that challenges your muscles as well as your breathing capability. Cardiovascular exercise is always a combination of the two: the ability of your body to take in oxygen, and the ability of your muscles to take up that oxygen and use it for the requirements of the exercise. So spend 15 seconds to gradually increase the resistance level to the point where your leg muscles feel challenged, as if you were riding up a fairly steep hill. This is in contrast to the practice of keeping the resistance low and increasing the revolutions per minute (rpm) at which you are cycling. For endurance training, the

1
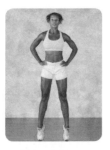

Squat Jump
Page 198
Cardio Interval:
Stationary bicycle

2
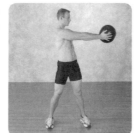

Standing Rotation With
Medicine Ball
See figure 4.12 on page 59

3
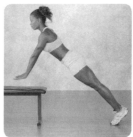

Plyometric Push-Up
Against Bench
Page 150
Cardio Interval:
Stationary bicycle

4
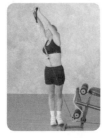

Reverse Chop With Cable
Page 172

5
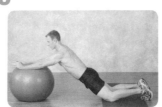

Lat Roll-Out on Stability Ball
Note: Focus on slowing
down the movement.
Page 144

6
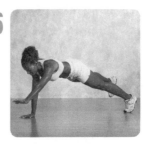

Crab Walk
Page 189
Cardio Interval:
Stationary bicycle

lower resistance would make sense, but in this workout for power, you want to increase the resistance and maintain a cadence of approximately 80 rpm. After you reach the right level and find your cadence in the first 15 seconds, you will do intervals at a work to rest ratio of 1:1. This means that for every interval of work, you will "rest" for the same amount of time. In this workout you will ride hard for 30 seconds and then ride easier for 30 seconds, catching your breath. You will do this three times for a total of 3 1/4 minutes—15 seconds to get your resistance, then three intervals of one minute each (30 seconds hard and 30 seconds easier). Remember, during the hard part of the interval, the resistance should be challenging enough to make you feel that it's difficult to continue. During the rest phase, you should set the resistance at a level that allows you to catch your breath enough to work intensely again in the next interval.

Do this entire series three times. Then do the body-weight and core exercises (exercise numbers 6-9) three times each, with a cardio interval in between each set. Refer to chapter 5 for guidelines on choosing weight for power routines. Do 3 to 10 repetitions of each exercise.

7

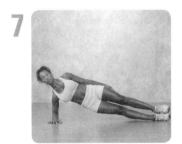

Lateral Hold on Forearm
Page 176
Cardio Interval:
Stationary bicycle

8

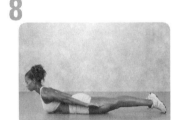

Back Extension
Page 185
Cardio Interval:
Stationary bicycle

9

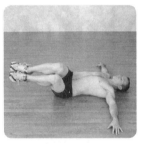

Supine Rotation
Note: **Do as quickly as**
safely possible.
Page 184

45-Minute Workout for General Health and Fitness

When you are working out to improve your general health and fitness, you can take the time for a longer warm-up and incorporate more cardio intervals into your routine. So pick two warm-ups instead of one from chapter 4. This routine is a good choice for a morning workout if you realize that you won't have time later in the day to do a cardio workout; it lets you address more of your fitness needs in one workout. When jumping rope, if you mess up, start again and keep going until you have accrued one minute of actual jumping time.

Do this routine twice. Chapter 5 gives you guidelines on choosing weight for routines for general health and fitness. Do 8 to 12 repetitions of each exercise.

1

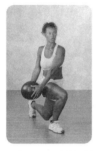

Walking Lunge With Rotation and Medicine Ball
Page 202
Cardio Interval: **Jump rope for 1 minute**

2

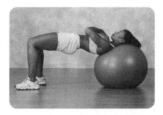

Bridge With Upper Body on Stability Ball
Page 209

3

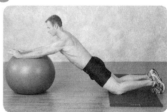

Lat Roll-Out on Stability Ball
Page 144
Cardio Interval: **Jump rope for 1 minute**

4

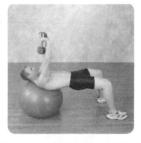

Pull-Over With Dumbbell on Stability Ball
Page 143

5

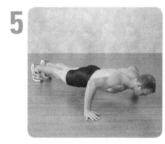

Walking Push-Up
Page 148

6

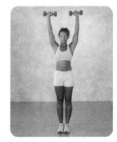

Standing Shoulder Press With Dumbbells
Note: **Alternate arms.**
Page 157

7

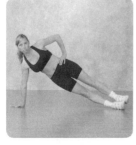

Lateral Hold With Straight Arm
Page 177

8

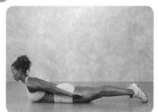

Back Extension
Page 185

9

60-Minute Programs

||||||||||||||||||||||||||||||||||||||||||||||||||||||||||||||||||||||||||||||||||||||||||||||||||||||||||||||||

Having a full 60 minutes to work out in the morning means that you can address various elements of fitness in a single routine. These workouts challenge your stability, balance, core strength, and cardiovascular fitness along with your strength. If you can take the time to do them, you'll be able to reap the benefits of a truly integrated strength program, improving your health in so many ways—and efficiently, too!

60-Minute Workout for Strength

Since you have time for some extra sets with the 60-minute workout, try to get the weight so challenging that it is literally impossible for you to lift it more than eight times. When you're working this hard, you will want to rest 30 to 60 seconds after each set to catch your breath and replenish your muscular energy.

1

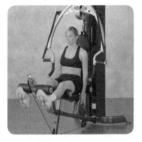

Squat With Barbell
Page 195

2

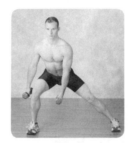

Single-Leg Squat With Opposite-Arm Reach
Page 197

3

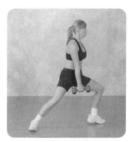

Leg Press
Page 214

4

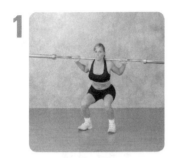

Leg Extension
Page 216

5

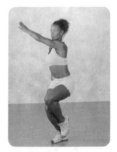

Lateral Lunge With Dumbbells
Page 203

6

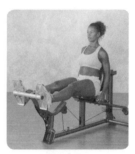

Rotation Lunge With Dumbbells
Page 204

7

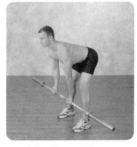

Deadlift With Barbell
Page 207

8

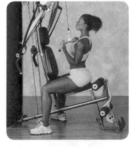

Lat Pull-Down
Page 140

9

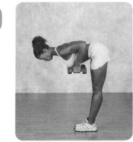

Unsupported Row With Dumbbells
Page 136

Refer to chapter 5 for more information about how much weight to use for strength workouts. Do two or three sets of each exercise with 30 to 60 seconds rest in between, and 7 or 8 repetitions of each exercise per set.

10
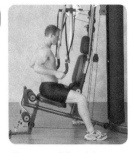
**Row on Machine
Page 139**

11
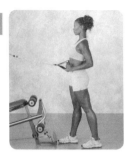
**Row With Cable
Page 138**

12
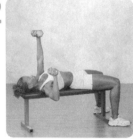
**Alternating Chest Press
With Dumbbells on Bench
Page 152**

13
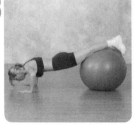
**Push-Up With Legs
on Stability Ball
Page 149**

14
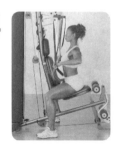
**Horizontal Row on Machine
Page 164**

15
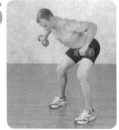
**Standing Horizontal Row
With Dumbbells
Page 160**

16
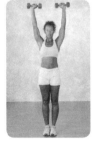
**Standing Shoulder Press
With Dumbbells
Page 157**

17
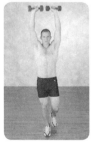
**Single-Leg Standing Biceps
Curl Into Shoulder Press
With Dumbbells
Page 158**

60-Minute Workout for Size

This routine will challenge your balance with exercises that require you to stand on one leg for a moment before continuing the movement. It's great to be able to incorporate this important element into your full-body morning routine, instead of having to take the time for a separate exercise that just addresses your balance.

1

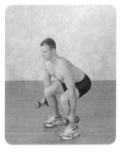

**Free-Standing Squat
With Dumbbells
Page 194**

2

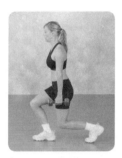

**Reverse Lunge With Dumbbells
Note: Stand on one leg 2 to 3
seconds between each lunge.
Page 200**

3

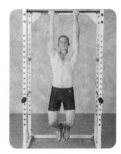

**Negative Chin-Up
Page 145**

4

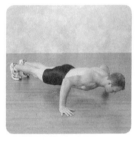

**Walking Push-Up
Page 148**

5

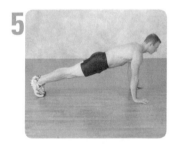

**Prone Hold on Hands
Page 175**

6

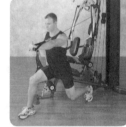

**Standing Single-Arm Chest
Press and Lunge With Cable
Page 155**

7

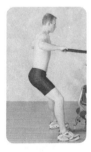

**Horizontal Row With Cable
Note: Stand on right leg for half
of set, left leg for rest of set.
Page 161**

8

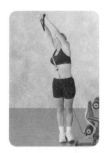

**Reverse Chop With Cable
Page 172**

9

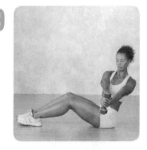

**Seated Rotation
With Dumbbell
Page 179**

Circuit 1 is composed of exercises 1 through 9, and circuit 2 is composed of exercises 10 through 17. Each circuit is a full-body routine; do each circuit two times. Refer to chapter 5 for information on how to pick the correct weight for routines that develop size. Do 10 to 15 repetitions of each exercise.

10
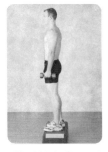

Step-Up With Dumbbells
Note: Balance on one foot for 2 to 3 seconds between steps.
Page 206

11
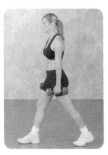

Walking Lunge With Dumbbells
Note: Stand on one leg 2 to 3 seconds between each lunge.
Page 201

12
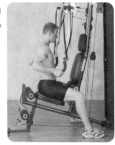

Row on Machine
Note: Alternate arms.
Page 139

13
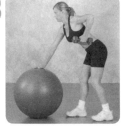

Single-Arm Row With Dumbbell on Stability Ball
Page 135

14
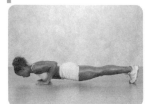

Push-Up
Page 146

15
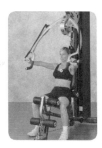

Seated Chest Press on Machine
Note: Alternate arms.
Page 156

16
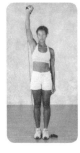

Standing Single-Arm Shoulder Press with Tubing
Page 159

17
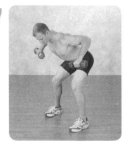

Standing Horizontal Row With Dumbbells
Note: Alternate arms.
Page 160

60-Minute Workout for Endurance

This routine starts with an extended core challenge, targeting the muscles in your midsection. It is therefore a great choice if you want to work those muscles more, or if you perhaps missed your Pilates workout this week. Pilates exercises involve numerous movements that focus on the muscles of your midsection and help stabilize your spine. Pilates programs have become very popular the last few years.

1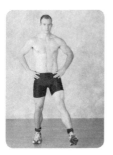

Band Walking
Page 211

2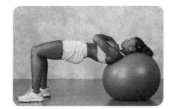

Bridge With Upper Body
on Stability Ball
Page 209

3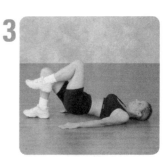

Single-Leg Bridge on Floor
Page 210

4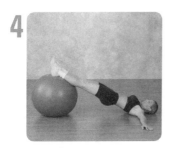

Bridge With Lower Body on
Stability Ball
Page 208

5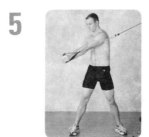

Standing Chop With Cable
Page 190

6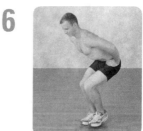

Single-Leg Squat
Page 196

7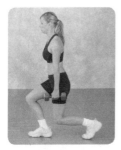

Reverse Lunge With Dumbbells
Note: Stand on one leg 2 to 3
seconds between each lunge.
Page 200

8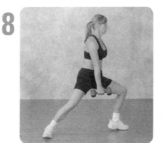

Clock Lunge with Dumbbells
Note: Variation of Rotation
Lunge With Dumbbells.
Page 204

9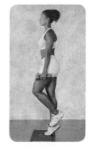

Single-Leg Heel Raise
With Dumbbell
Page 212

Chapter 5 gives detailed information on how to pick the correct weight for your endurance routines. Do the entire sequence three times, and do 15 to 25 repetitions of each exercise.

10
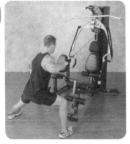
Standing Lateral Lunge With Single-Arm Horizontal Row and Cable
Page 163

11
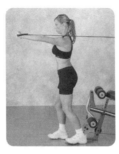
Standing Single-Arm Chest Press With Tubing
Page 154

12
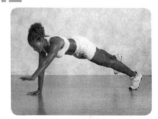
Crab Walk
Note: Do slowly.
Page 189

13
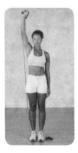
Standing Single-Arm Shoulder Press With Tubing
Page 159

14
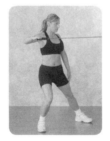
Standing Lateral Lunge With Single-Arm Horizontal Row and Tubing
Page 162

60-Minute Workout for Power

Since by definition you aren't able to do many repetitions when you're working really hard, this routine incorporates some high-intensity cardio intervals. Take as much time as you need to catch your breath between exercises. This will give you a chance to recover so that you can work hard again. This workout uses a stationary bicycle for the cardio intervals (you can substitute a treadmill or elliptical machine if you need to). Refer to the 45-minute power workout on page 114 for information about cardio intervals.

1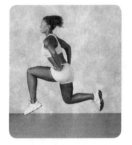

Jump Lunge
Page 205
Cardio Interval: Stationary
bicycle

2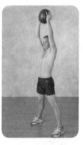

Squat With Medicine Ball Lift
See figure 4.10 on page 58
Note: Squat slowly, and lift
the ball overhead quickly.

3

Plyometric Push-Up
Against Bench
Page 150
Cardio Interval:
Stationary bicycle

4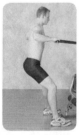

Horizontal Row With Cable
Note: Do relatively quickly.
Page 161

5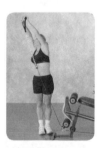

Reverse Chop With Cable
Page 172
Cardio Interval:
Stationary bicycle

6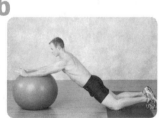

Lat Roll-Out on Stability Ball
Note: Focus on slowing down
the movement; hold for 5
seconds.
Page 144

Refer to chapter 5 for recommendations on how much weight to use in routines aimed at developing power. Do this entire series three times, with 3 to 10 repetitions of each exercise per set. Then do the body-weight and core exercises three times each.

7

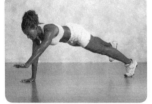

Crab Walk *Note:* **Move side to side for one minute.**
Page 189
Cardio Interval:
Stationary bicycle

8

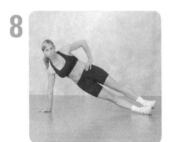

Lateral Hold With Straight Arm
Page 177

9

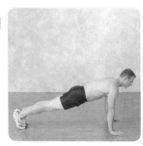

Prone Hold on Hands
Page 175
Cardio Interval:
Stationary bicycle

10

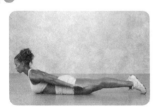

Back Extension
Page 185

11

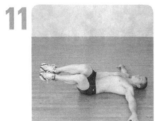

Supine Rotation
Note: **Do as quickly as safely possible.**
Page 184
Cardio Interval:
Stationary bicycle

12

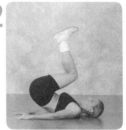

Reverse Crunch
Page 183

60-Minute Workout for General Health and Fitness

Pick a longer warm-up to do before getting started on this routine. This will be beneficial if your goal is to improve your general health and fitness, since the warm-ups in this book address various elements of fitness for a well-rounded program. This routine incorporates cardio intervals into the workout; you can use either a treadmill, stationary bike, or elliptical machine to do these.

1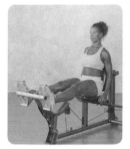

Leg Press
Page 214

2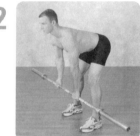

Deadlift With Barbell
Page 207
Cardio Interval: 3 minutes on treadmill, stationary bicycle, or elliptical machine

3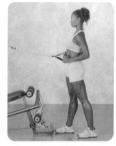

Row With Cable
Note: Pull from below.
Page 138

4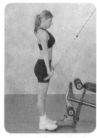

Straight-Arm Pull-Down With Cable
Page 141

5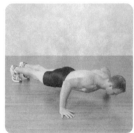

Walking Push-Up
Page 148
Cardio Interval: 3 minutes on treadmill, stationary bicycle, or elliptical machine

6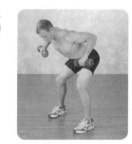

Standing Horizontal Row With Dumbbells
Page 160

Refer to chapter 5 for recommendations on the weight that you should use for workouts for general health and fitness. Do this entire sequence twice, with 8 to 12 repetitions of each exercise unless otherwise noted.

7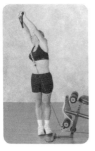

Reverse Chop With Cable
Page 172

8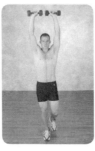

Single-Leg Standing Biceps Curl Into Shoulder Press With Dumbbells
Page 158

9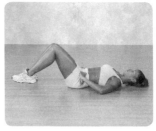

Toe Tap
Note: **Do for 1 minute.**
Page 169
Cardio Interval: **3 minutes on treadmill, stationary bicycle, or elliptical machine**

Morning Exercises

10

Upper Body

|||||||||||||||||||||||||||||||||||||||||||||||||||||||||||||||||||||||||||||||||||||||||||||||||||||||||||||||||||||||||||||||||||||||

Most upper-body exercises involve moving your arms at your shoulder or elbow joints (or both together). These joints and the muscles that operate them can perform a wide variety of movements that you can incorporate into your morning strength workout. Here is some information about your shoulder girdle, shoulder joint, and your elbow.

- **Shoulder girdle.** Your shoulder girdle is made up of your scapulae, both of your clavicle bones, and your sternum (breastbone). The shoulder girdle is very important in upper-body exercises, because it works in unison with your shoulder joint and stabilizes the movement, enabling you to lift more weight. The movements at your shoulder girdle include elevation, lifting your shoulder blades up, and depression, pulling them down. Retraction means pulling your shoulder blades together, and protraction is pulling them apart. When you use your shoulders in exercise, you can improve their performance by visualizing your shoulder girdle and your shoulder joint moving together in a smooth rhythm. For example, when you do a push-up, you should feel how your shoulder blades gently separate as you push away from the floor and then move toward each other again as you lower your body.

- **Shoulder joint.** Your shoulder joint is made up of the humerus (the bone of your upper arm) and the scapula (shoulder blade). The top end of the humerus fits into the glenoid fossa (shallow indentation) of the scapula. It can do many different kinds of movements, including flexion, which is when you lift your arm up in front of you, and extension, which is when you pull your arm down or back from the front. The shoulder joint can also abduct your arm, bringing it out to the side and up toward the ceiling, and adduct it, bringing it from the side down toward your body. The joint can abduct and adduct the arm along the transverse (horizontal) plane as well. These motions begin with your arm held out to the side, at shoulder height; bringing the arm forward from this position is horizontal adduction, and bringing it back behind you is horizontal abduction. Finally, the shoulder joint can rotate your entire arm internally (inward) and externally (outward).

• **Elbow.** Your elbow has two basic motions: It can flex the arm, decreasing the distance between your upper arm and your forearm, and it can extend the arm, essentially straightening it at the elbow. You can also rotate around the elbow. If you bend your elbow to 90 degrees, you can rotate your forearm so that your thumb turns out and the palm of your hand faces the ceiling. This is called supination. The opposite movement, where you turn your thumb to the inside and your palm faces the floor is called pronation.

The exercises in this chapter are designed to target more than one muscle at a time. This makes for very efficient morning sessions, because you get more of a workout by challenging multiple muscles simultaneously than by challenging just one at a time. This approach is also more functional, meaning that the exercises simulate real life, in which you use several different muscles in unison. Some of the muscles that the upper-body exercises in this chapter target are:

• **Latissimus Dorsi.** Your latissimus dorsi (lat muscle) starts at the deep lumbar fascia of your low back and comes up at a diagonal angle on each side, covering much of the back. It then comes up underneath your shoulders and attaches to the front of your upper arms. Whenever you do an exercise in which you pull toward your body from either the front or the side, you are working your lats. When you do a row, your lats pull your arms back from the front (shoulder extension). When you pull your arms down from the sides, as in a lateral pull-down, you are using your lats to do shoulder adduction. Your lats also internally rotate your shoulders. This can sometimes contribute to postural problems if you don't balance out your program or if you use improper form and let your shoulders round forward a lot as you do the exercises. Always remember to keep your shoulders down and back as you do any exercise.

• **Pectoralis Major.** The pectoralis major muscle group starts along your clavicle and sternum. From these bones, the muscle fibers cross your chest and attach to the front of your upper arm. Depending on which angle you are working from, your pectoralis major can perform several movements. One of these that is frequent in our workouts is pulling your arms together at about shoulder height; this is called horizontal adduction. Along with the lats, the pec major also helps bring about internal rotation, making them another potential cause of the internally rotated posture we see so often in the gym and everyday life. This posture can result from strengthening the pecs too much relative to the opposing muscles of the upper-middle back or from sustaining a position for a long time, such as when working at a desk. To avoid developing this posture, be sure to work the muscles of the upper-middle back equally with the pecs.

The upper-body exercises in this book that target your pecs work your anterior deltoids and triceps at the same time. Again, this approach is more efficient than exercise plans that isolate each individual muscle.

• **Deltoids.** The deltoid, or shoulder muscle, is divided into three sections: anterior (front), medial (middle), and posterior (rear). When you stand with your arm relaxed at your side, its fibers run more or less up and down. Depending on which way you move your arm against gravity, you can target one section more than another. The anterior fibers flex your arm at the shoulder, bringing it up and forward from a position of resting at your side, and also horizontally adduct your arm, bringing it forward from a position of being held out to the side, parallel to the floor. The medial fibers abduct your arm, lifting it out to the side and overhead. The posterior deltoids do the opposite of the anterior fibers—they extend your arm, pulling it backward from a flexed or resting position, and horizontally abduct your arm, pulling it back from the position of being held up parallel to the floor.

• **Triceps.** The word *triceps* means "three heads." The long head of the muscle starts on your scapula, which means it also contributes to shoulder extension. The other two heads start on the humerus. The entire muscle attaches to the ulna, which is one of the bones of the forearm. The main function of the triceps is to extend, or straighten out, the elbow.

• **Shoulder girdle muscles.** The muscles of your shoulder girdle do not contribute directly to the movement at the shoulder joint, but they do work together with the joint. These muscles include the rhomboids, which pull the scapulae toward the spine, and the trapezius, which is divided into three sections, each with its own function. The upper trapezius elevates, or shrugs, your shoulder; the middle trapezius adducts, or pulls together, your scapulae; and the lower trapezius depresses, or pulls down, the scapulae. Many of us have upper trapezius muscles that are too tight or just overactive. When you perform any of the exercises in this chapter that require you to contract your trapezius, be sure to keep your shoulder blades down and back, without straining.

It is really important to work the muscles of your upper-middle back and the back of your shoulders more often than your pecs and anterior deltoids, since work habits (like hunching over in front of a computer) and gravity itself often contribute to a posture that is too rounded forward. For this reason, the workouts in this book emphasize the posterior muscles more than the anterior ones.

Single-Arm Row With Dumbbell on Bench

This targets your lat muscle, as well as your arm. It also challenges your core strength, which you need to hold your body still on the bench. Stand just to the right of the bench. Place your left knee and left hand on the bench, far enough apart to get your spine in a neutral position, with your chest out and your shoulders down and back. Hold the dumbbell in your right hand, with your right arm pointing straight down toward the floor (1). Exhale as you pull your right elbow up toward the ceiling, keeping it close to your side (2). Think of pulling your shoulder blades down and back as you move your arm. Look toward the floor to keep your neck neutral. Repeat on the other side.

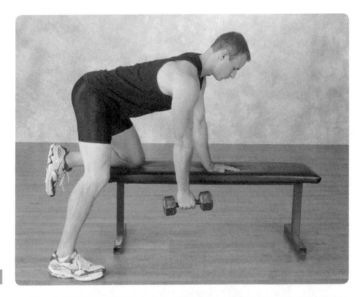

1

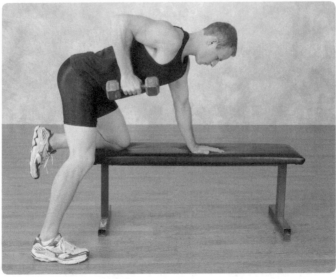

2

Single-Arm Row With Dumbbell on Stability Ball

This also targets your lat muscle and your arm. Holding your body still as you perform the row challenges your core strength even more than the previous exercise, since the ball is unstable. Stand with the stability ball a little in front of you and to your right. Place your right hand on the ball as you lean forward from your hips, keeping your chest out and your shoulders down and back. Hold the dumbbell in your left hand, with your left arm pointing straight down toward the floor (1). Exhale as you pull your left elbow up toward the ceiling, keeping it close to your side (2). Think of pulling your shoulder blades down and back as you move your arm. Look toward the floor to keep your neck neutral. Repeat on the other side.

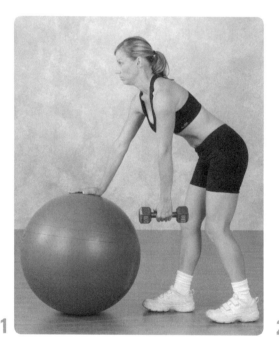

1

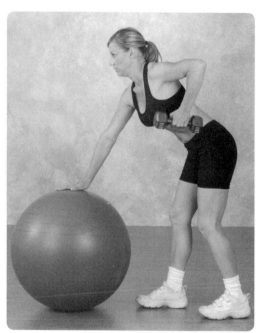

2

Unsupported Row With Dumbbells

This targets your lats and your arms, and it's more challenging to your core muscles, since you have to hold yourself up instead of using equipment such as a bench for support. When doing an exercise like this, you need to flex from your hips to align yourself correctly against gravity as you lift the dumbbell. Many people have a hard time distinguishing between flexing from the hips and flexing from the spine. To get an idea of the posture that you want, stand with your right side facing a mirror and notice the natural curve in your low back. Now, lean forward from your hips, making sure the curve in your low back does not decrease—you want to avoid letting your low back curl forward.

Take a dumbbell in each hand and hold them by your sides. Lean forward from your hips until you cannot go any farther without losing your neutral spine. (If your hamstrings are tight you may not be able to lean very far forward, but it gets easier with practice.) This is your starting position (1). Let your arms hang down perpendicular to the floor. Face the floor to keep your neck neutral. As you exhale, pull your elbows up toward the ceiling, keeping them close to your sides (2). Pull your shoulder blades down and back as you do the movement.

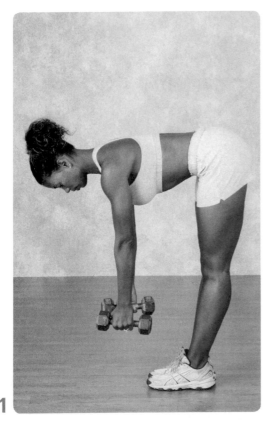

1

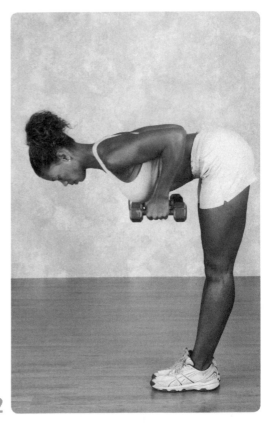

2

Row With Tubing

This targets your lats and your arms. When using tubing, you can add variety by changing the angles you pull from. Loop the tubing around a stable object that faces you. You can change the angle from which you pull by putting the tubing at different heights. It can be placed high, above your shoulders, so that you are essentially pulling down, or it can be low so that you are pulling up. You can also place the tubing at chest height. Holding one grip in each hand, step back far enough to feel some tension in the tubing before you start, and try to get equal resistance on both sides. Stand with your feet hip-width apart (1). As you exhale, bend your elbows and pull them back, keeping them close to your body, and pull your shoulders down and back (2). If you want to feel more stable doing the exercise, you can stagger your feet, putting one foot a little in front of the other. If you do this, however, be sure to keep both feet facing straight ahead.

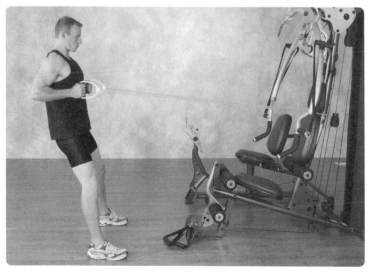

1

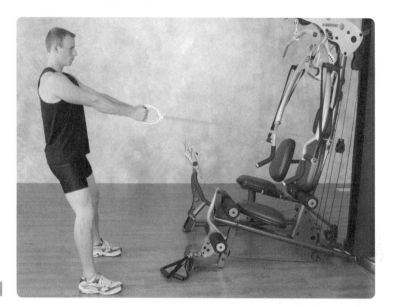

2

Row With Cable

This targets your lats and your arms. There are many kinds of cable equipment available. The newer styles have not only adjustable cable heights but also more freely moving pulleys and cams around which the cables move. This gives you the opportunity to perform rows from all different angles, allowing you to vary your program to constantly challenge your body. You can adjust the cable to whatever height you like.

Grip the cable handles with one or both hands. Stand far enough away from the cable column to get some resistance before you start the exercise. If you want to feel more stable, you can stagger your feet, putting one foot a little in front of the other. Keep both feet facing straight ahead (1). As you exhale, pull your arms back, keeping your elbows close to your body. Pull your shoulders down and back as you do the exercise (2). Vary your routine from session to session (e.g., pull from straight ahead, then next time pull from the top, and next from the bottom). You can also row with one arm, you can rotate slightly in the direction of that arm as you row, and you can alternate arms.

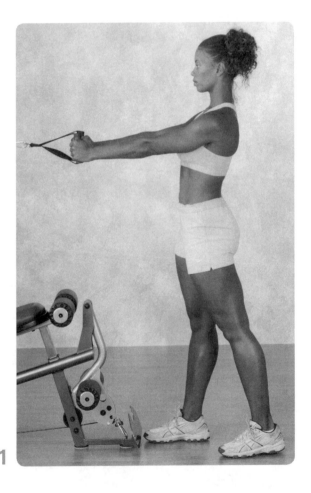

1

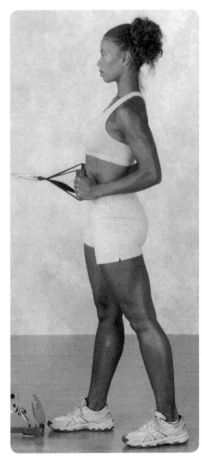

2

Row on Machine

This targets your lats and your arms. To figure out how high the seat should be, do the rowing movement without holding the grips. Begin by sitting on the machine facing the pad and holding your arms straight out in front of you, with your thumbs up. Bend your elbows and pull your arms back, keeping them close to your body. Then, when you perform the row holding on to the vertical grips, you should get the same movement pattern, without your forearms going higher or lower than before. If the seat is too high, you will notice that you flex your elbow a lot when doing the movement. If the seat is too low, you'll have trouble bending your elbows even to 90 degrees. Experiment and adjust the seat accordingly.

When doing a machine row, try to sit up straight and tall and use your core muscles to stabilize your body, without leaning into the chest pad too much. Keep your feet flat on the floor. Adjust the chest pad before you begin so that you have to reach forward a little bit to get the grips. To do the row, hold on to the grips with palms facing each other and thumbs pointing toward the ceiling (1). As you exhale, pull your shoulders down and back as you pull your elbows back, keeping them close to your body (2).

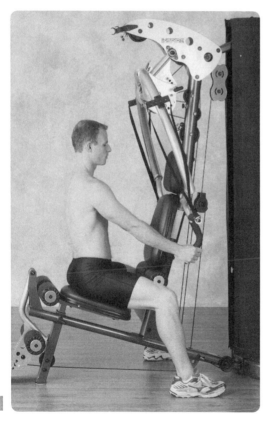

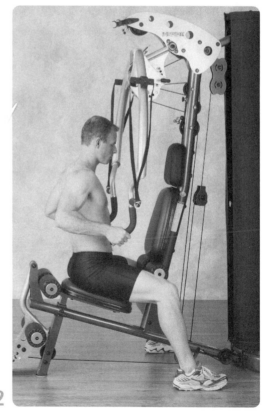

1

2

Lat Pull-Down

This works the latissimus dorsi, posterior deltoids, and biceps. When you do a lat (lateral) pull-down using an underhand grip so that your arms come down from the front next to your body, you're doing shoulder extension, just like in the row exercise. When you hold the bar with an overhand grip and pull down so your elbows go out to the sides, you're doing shoulder adduction. Holding the bar with an underhand grip targets your biceps a little more, since it's your biceps that help bring about the movement of supination (turning your forearm and fist out). You can alternate the type of lat pull-down exercise you do, using an underhand grip for one session and for the next session using an overhand grip with your arms bending to the side as they come down.

Seated at the lat pull-down machine, grab the bar, hands a little farther apart than shoulder width (1). If you want to work your core muscles as well as your upper body, do not use the pad for your thighs. As you exhale, pull your shoulder blades down and back, and pull your elbows down and to your sides (2). Stop when your elbows get to your sides. It does not matter where the bar ends up.

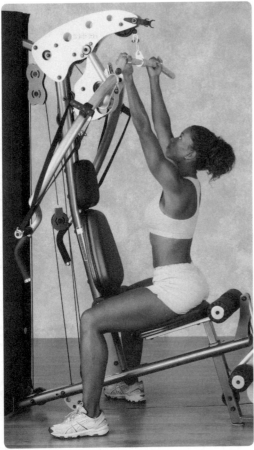

1

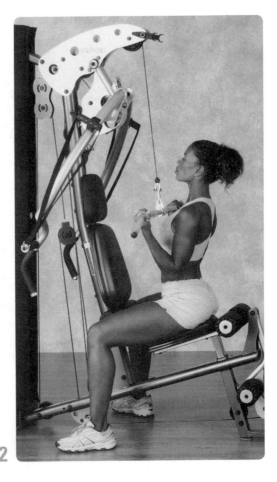

2

Straight-Arm Pull-Down With Cable

This exercise targets your lats and your triceps, along with your posterior deltoids. It's also great for your core since you have to stand up and hold yourself still as you do the exercise. Set the cable up so that it is coming from the top of the cable column. Use either a straight bar or two individual grips from the same cable. Stand far enough away so that you feel tension in the cable and the plates you are using are lifted, not touching the rest of the stack, when your arms and body are positioned to begin the exercise. Hold your arms up and lean forward from your hips to align yourself with the way the cable is being pulled (1). As you exhale, pull your shoulder blades down and together as you bring your arms down to your sides so they end right next to your body (2).

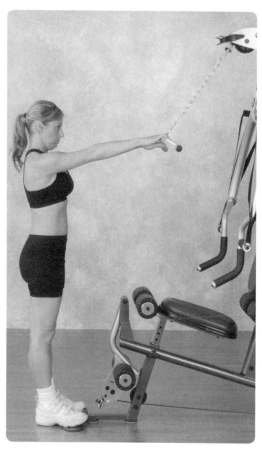

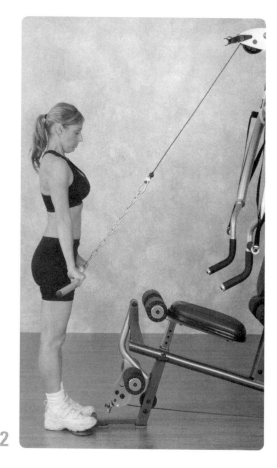

1

2

Pull-Over With Dumbbell on Bench

A pull-over exercise involves shoulder extension just as the row does, but it is different for a couple of reasons. Because you are lying down when you perform the pull-over, you need to use your core muscles to stabilize your body as you move the dumbbell. Also, you start with your arms stretched out behind your head (so that if you were standing, they would be pointing up to the ceiling) and the dumbbell perpendicular to gravity, which makes it feel relatively heavy. Then, you stop the movement when the dumbbell is lifted directly above the body.

Sit on a bench with one foot on each side. Grasp a dumbbell with both hands and hold it at your midsection with the ends pointing up and down. Lie back on the bench. You can bring your feet up, putting both feet on the bench with your knees bent, or you can keep your feet on the floor. You can make the exercise more challenging to your core if you lift up one or both feet while you perform it. Bring the dumbbell behind your head so that your arms are stretched out in line with your body (if you were upright, they would be reaching over your head toward the ceiling). They should be relatively straight at the elbows (1). As you exhale, pull your shoulder blades down and back and lift the dumbbell up over your head and chest until your arms are perpendicular to your body (2).

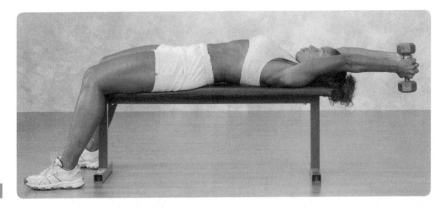

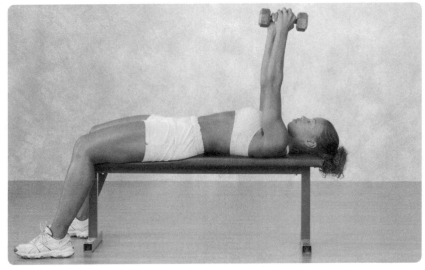

Pull-Over With Dumbbell on Stability Ball

Using a stability ball instead of a bench requires you to use your core muscles more to balance and stabilize the exercise since the ball is an unstable surface. You will not be able to lift as much weight as you can when you use a bench, so this variation is a good choice for your endurance workouts, when you're working with a relatively light weight. The stability ball you use should be big enough so that your thighs are more or less parallel to the floor when you sit down on it.

After you sit down, hold the dumbbell at your midsection with the ends pointing straight up and down, and walk your feet forward, allowing your body to gradually lie back on the ball. Walk far enough to get your shoulders and head on the ball, keeping your neck in a neutral position at all times. Bring the dumbbell up over and behind your head so that your arms are stretched out behind you parallel to the floor, keeping your elbows relatively straight (1). As you exhale, pull your shoulder blades down and back and lift your arms up over your head and chest until they are perpendicular to your body (2).

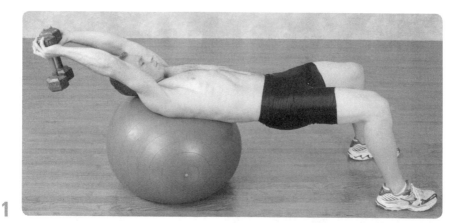

1

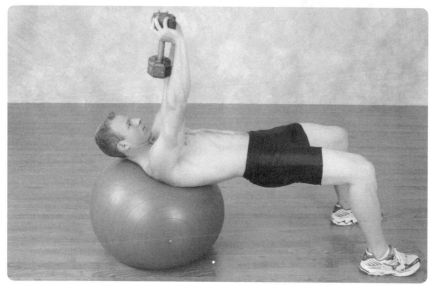

2

Lat Roll-Out on Stability Ball

This exercise works your lats in a shoulder extension movement—that is, you are pulling your arms down (relative to your body) to your sides. It also challenges your posterior deltoids, triceps, and core as well as your shoulder girdle stability. Kneel facing the stability ball and put your hands on top of it, with your palms down and arms no more than shoulder-width apart (1). The bigger the ball, the easier this exercise will be, since you are farther away from the floor. Lean forward about 20 degrees, moving at your knees and keeping your spine neutral. The ball will roll forward as your body leans closer to the floor, hinging at your knees (2). Your arms stay relatively still as you do the movement, but keep your elbows soft. Reverse the motion and pull back. The farther you roll out, the more difficult this exercise becomes. Be sure to keep your spine neutral the entire time, and only roll out as far as you can maintain it. If you do this exercise with a mirror to one side, you'll get good feedback as to your form.

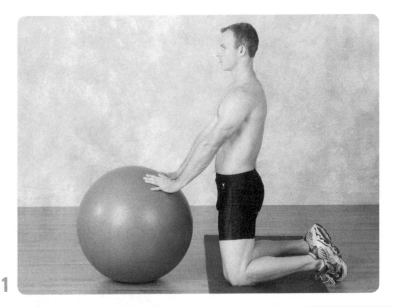

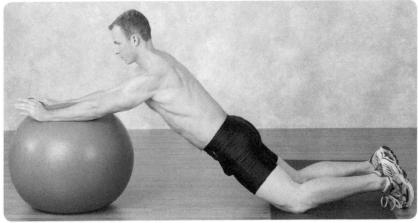

Chin-Up

Many of us are relatively weak in our upper body and core, making a chin-up a very difficult exercise because it requires pulling your entire body up away from gravity. Chin-ups are performed with an underhand grip on the bar. They work your lats and your biceps. Your biceps work especially hard in this underhand grip since it puts your forearm in a position of supination, where your palm is rotated out.

Start by hanging on the bar. You might need to get a stool or a bench to help you get up to the starting position. Hold on to the bar with your arms about shoulder-width apart (1). Pull your shoulder blades down and back as you pull yourself up. Pull up until your elbows are bent and at your sides, with your chin close to the bar (2).

If you cannot pull yourself up, you can do a negative chin-up instead. This means that you climb up to the end position at the top, and then lower yourself slowly. Do this by using a chair or a bench so that you can get high enough to start at the top position. Lowering yourself is easier than lifting yourself up because you are working toward gravity instead of away from it, and also because your muscles have less internal friction when they are lengthening than when they are shortening. Doing negative chin-ups is a great way to develop strength!

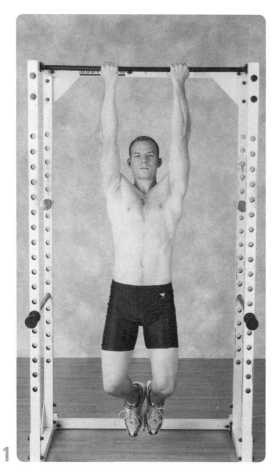
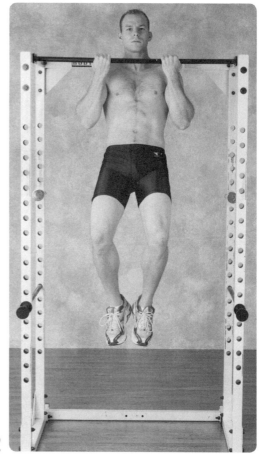

1

2

Push-Up

Like the chin-up, the push-up is a wonderful exercise since it makes you move your own body away from gravity. It is a challenge for your core and upper body. A push-up challenges your pecs and anterior deltoids, and also your triceps, since you have to straighten your arms out at the elbows.

Lie facedown on a mat or on the floor. Put your hands on the surface, placing your palms nearly under your shoulders but a little farther apart than shoulder width and just a little farther back toward your midsection. Now straighten your arms and lift your body from your toes, keeping your spine neutral in your low back and neck so that your body forms a straight line from your toes or knees to the top of your head (1). From this position, lower yourself to where your elbows are at 90 degrees or less, maintaining that straight line throughout your body (2), and then push back up. You can also do push-ups from your knees (3, 4).

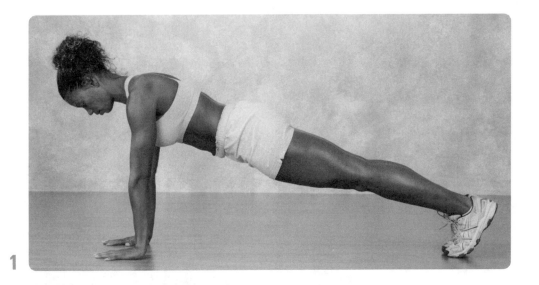

1

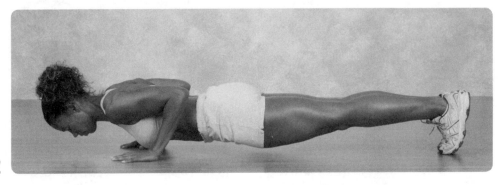

2

You can do push-ups at any angle. The more upright the angle of your body, the easier it will be, because your center of gravity will be lower and less weight will fall on your arms. You can start by doing push-ups against a wall and move on to more challenging positions by doing them against a bench or bar at progressively lower heights. Another variable that you can change very easily is the position of your hands. If you place them asymmetrically—for example, keeping your right hand two inches (about five centimeters) farther forward than your left when you are working on the floor or two inches higher when you're working against the wall—it will put a different demand on your muscles and add dynamism to your workout.

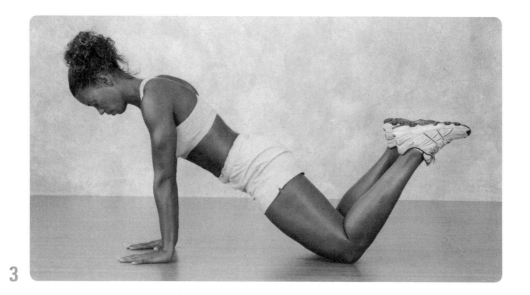

3

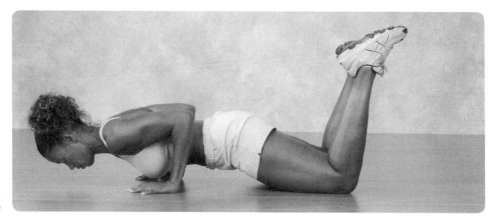

4

Walking Push-Up

This is a progression from the asymmetrical position described in the previous exercise. In this push-up, after each repetition you change the location of both hands (moving just one at a time). The constantly changing positions increase the demand on your joints to control the movement. Changing the angle at which you move challenges your muscle fibers in slightly different ways, forcing them to adapt and helping you become stronger in the various positions.

Get into your push-up position either on the floor or against the wall and do one repetition. Now, lift up your left hand and move it two inches (about five centimeters) to the left. Lift up your right hand and move it the same distance to the left (1), and then do another push-up (2). Next move your right hand, then your left, two inches (again, about five centimeters) back to the center and do another push-up. Then move to the right of center, and then back again. Essentially you're "walking" back and forth a short distance between repetitions. As you move your hands, you should also pivot at either your toes or knees. You can also move your hands a couple of inches forward or back to change the angles even more.

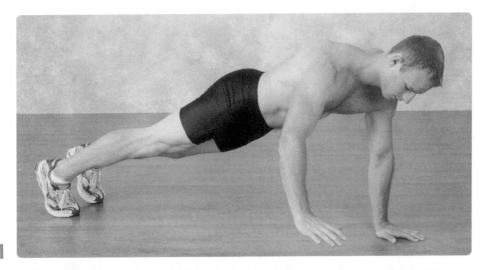

1

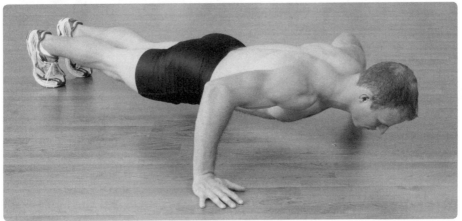

2

Push-Up With Legs on Stability Ball

This targets your pecs, anterior deltoids, and triceps, as well as your core, which has to work in order to keep your legs still on top of the ball. The exercise gets more difficult as the ball gets bigger, since your legs are farther away from the floor and more weight is directed toward the arms.

Kneel on the floor facing the ball. Roll yourself onto the ball and place your hands on the floor on the other side of it (1). Walk your hands forward as your body rolls over the ball. From this position, lower your upper body to the floor, keeping the back straight (2). The farther you go to reach your starting position, the more challenging the push-ups will be, so begin with most of your lower legs on the ball. In future workouts, you can modify your position as you get stronger.

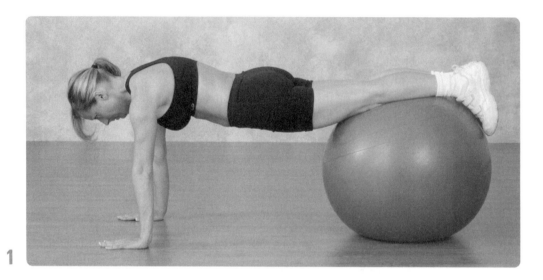

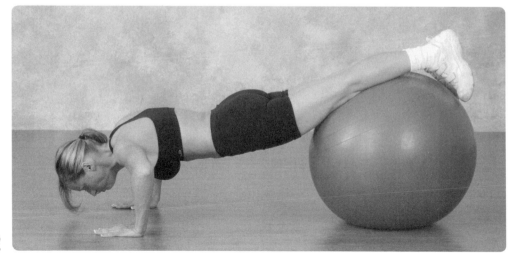

Plyometric Push-Up Against Bench

The term *plyometric* means a lengthening of the muscle fibers followed by a shortening of these fibers. The lengthening of the muscle fibers stores elastic energy, allowing for more powerful movement as the muscle fibers shorten again. The less time between the lengthening and the shortening phase, called the amortization phase, the more power you can produce. Incorporating plyometric movements into your workouts will improve your joint integrity, making your joints better able to withstand forces and quick changes of direction. Many people think that plyometric movements imply lots of weight or that they are only for elite athletes. This could not be further from the truth! The important thing is to find the appropriate level for you. If you try to do a plyometric push-up off the floor and you find you literally can't get up off the ground, then this type is too difficult for you—but you can do them against a wall or elevated surface, and your strength and stability will improve over time.

This exercise targets your pecs, anterior deltoids, and triceps. The plyometric force will also help improve the stability of your shoulders and arms. You can do this against a bench in the gym or on a park bench.

Put your hands on the bench, straighten your arms, and step back far enough to get your body in a straight line from your shoulders to your toes. Lower yourself halfway to the bench (1), then push away forcefully, so that your hands come up off the bench for a moment (2). As you come back toward the bench, slow the movement down, and then when you have lowered yourself halfway try to push away again relatively quickly.

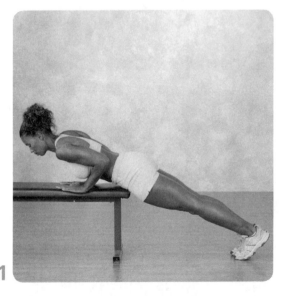

1

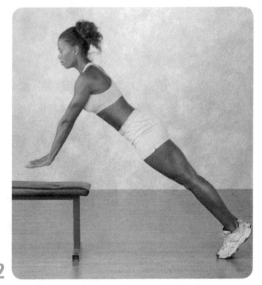

2

Chest Press With Dumbbells on Bench

Using dumbbells is harder than using a machine, since you have to control each hand individually. You also need to use your core more than when sitting on a machine. When you use a bench for this exercise, you can either keep your feet on the floor on either side or bring them up onto the bench with your knees bent and your feet flat. If you are able to keep your feet flat on the floor without losing your neutral spine, that is fine. If the bench is too high relative to the length of your legs, however, it's better to bring your feet up on the bench to do the exercise.

Start in the middle of the bench, holding a dumbbell in each hand. Lean back onto the bench, holding the weights close to your midsection until you feel secure in your position. Then bring the weights up so you are holding them straight above your body, shoulder-width apart. Position your hands with your palms facing forward. As you inhale, bend your elbows to 90 degrees out to the side so that your forearms are in straight lines, perpendicular to the floor (1). As you exhale, straighten out your arms, pushing the dumbbells up toward the ceiling and slightly toward each other (2).

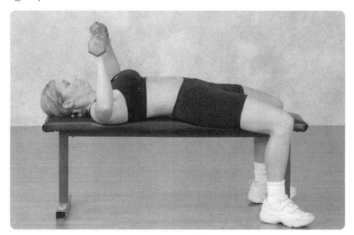

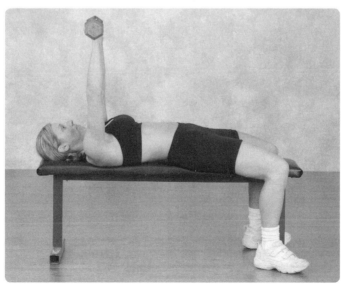

Alternating Chest Press With Dumbbells on Bench

For this exercise, you will alternate arms, keeping one in the ending position while performing another repetition with the other one and then switching sides. This puts more of a demand on your core to keep your body stable throughout the exercise. Start by sitting at the middle of the bench, holding a dumbbell in each hand. Lean back onto the bench, either bringing both feet up or keeping them on the floor. Hold the weights close to your midsection until you feel secure in your position. Then bring the weights up so you are holding them straight up above your body, shoulder-width apart. Hold your hands with your palms facing forward (1). As you inhale, bend your right elbow to 90 degrees out to the side so that your forearm is in a straight line, perpendicular to the floor (2). As you exhale, straighten out your arm, pushing the dumbbells up toward the ceiling and slightly toward each other. Hold your right arm there, and then bring only the left side down. Then on the next repetition, keep the left arm up, bringing the right arm down.

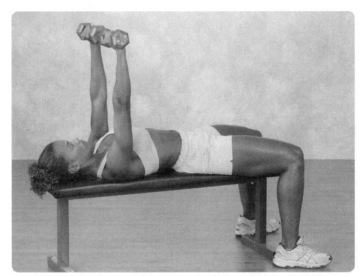

1

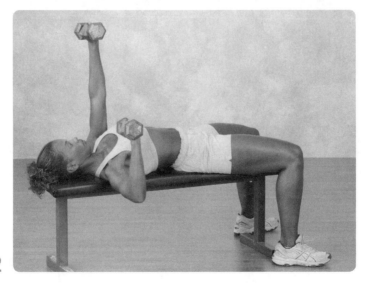

2

Chest Press With Dumbbells on Stability Ball

Just as with any exercise that uses a stability ball, you will have to work to stay stable and keep your balance throughout this exercise. You won't be able to lift as much weight as you can when using a bench or a chest-press machine, so this is a good choice when the main goal of your workout is to increase your muscles' endurance or size rather than strength or power. The stability ball should be big enough so that your thighs are more or less parallel to the floor when you sit on it. Sit on the ball with a dumbbell in each hand. Slowly walk your feet forward, holding the weights at your midsection and lying back onto the ball. Walk until your shoulders and head are resting on the ball, keeping your neck in a neutral position at all times.

Hold the weights close to your midsection until you feel secure in your position. Bring the weights up so you are holding them a few inches above your body around chest height. Push your arms straight up with your palms facing forward. Inhale, and bend your elbows out to the sides, to 90 degrees, so that your forearms are in straight lines, perpendicular to the floor (1). As you exhale, push the dumbbells up toward the ceiling and slightly toward each other (2).

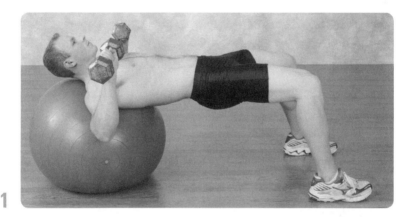

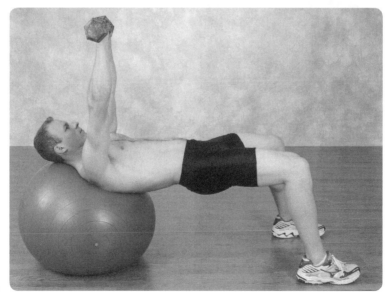

Standing Single-Arm Chest Press With Tubing

Wrap a piece of tubing around a stable object at about shoulder height. Take one grip of the tubing and put it through the grip at the other end to secure it. Stand facing away from the attached end of the tubing, and place your right leg in front of your left leg. Hold the free grip in your left hand, keeping it around chest height, with your elbow up and bent to about 90 degrees. Your arm should be about parallel to the floor, with your elbow pointing back (1). As you exhale, push forward with your left hand until your arm straightens out at the elbow (2). When you finish your repetitions, repeat on the opposite side.

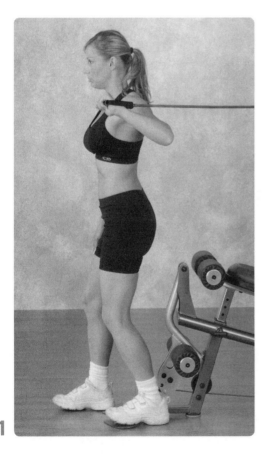

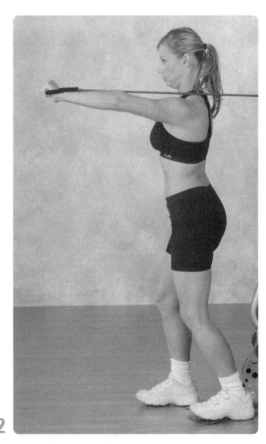

Standing Single-Arm Chest Press and Lunge With Cable

This targets your whole lower body, as well as your pecs, anterior deltoids, and triceps. Stand with both feet about hip-width apart, facing away from the source of the cable. Hold the single grip in your left hand, keeping it around chest height, with your elbow up and bent to about 90 degrees (1). As you exhale, step forward into a lunge with your right leg, and at the same time push forward with your left hand. Lunge until you get both knees bent to about 90 degrees (2). Then step back with your right leg, bringing your left arm back to the starting position. When you finish your repetitions, repeat on the opposite side.

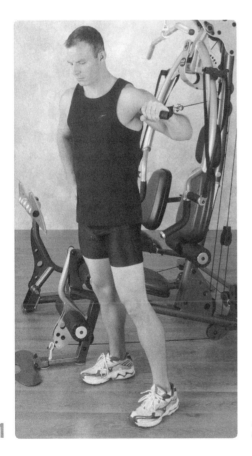

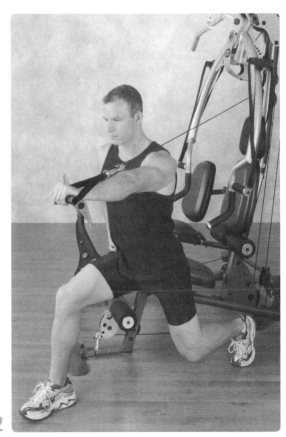

Seated Chest Press on Machine

This exercise targets your pectoralis major, anterior deltoids, and triceps. There are different types of chest-press machines; my instructions are based on the kind that is in most commercial health clubs. To determine the proper seat height, sit on the machine and hold your arms up so that your elbows are up, bent to about 90 degrees, and held out at approximately chest height. Your arms should be parallel to the floor. The height of the seat should be adjusted so that your arms are in this position when you hold the horizontal grips of the machine.

Hold on to the grips, and bring your arms back to where your elbows are alongside your body or slightly behind it (1). Push both arms or just one arm forward until your elbows are relatively straight (2). Doing the exercise with one arm challenges your core more to hold your body still.

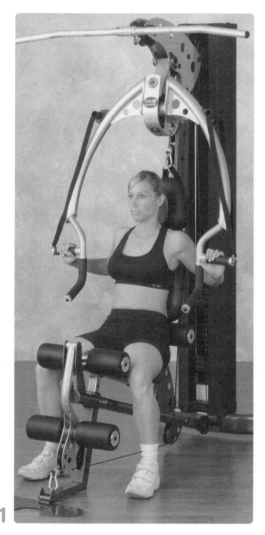 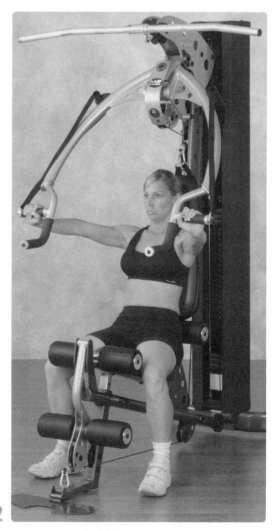

1　　　　　　　　2

Standing Shoulder Press With Dumbbells

This exercise targets your medial deltoids and triceps. Pick up the dumbbells and stand with your feet hip-width apart, or with one foot a little in front of the other in a staggered stance. This will give you more stability, but for a greater challenge, you can stand with your feet together. Hold the dumbbells up with your elbows bent to about 90 degrees and out to the side at shoulder height. Your forearms should be straight up and down with palms facing forward (1). As you exhale, push the weights up so that your arms straighten out (2). Lower them to where your elbows are again at about shoulder height.

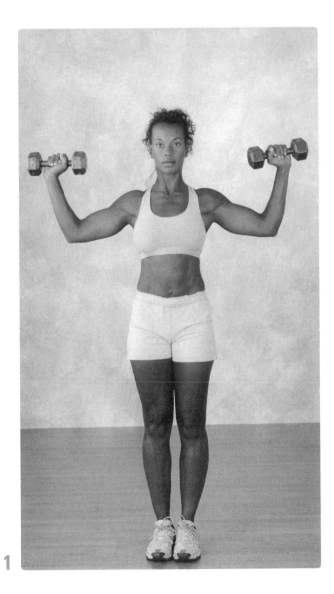

1

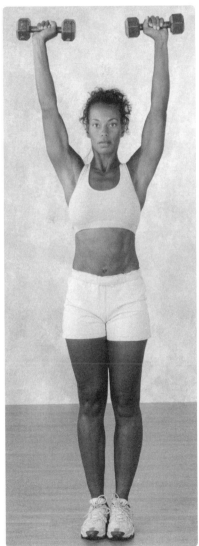

2

Single-Leg Standing Biceps Curl Into Shoulder Press With Dumbbells

This targets your medial deltoids, triceps, and biceps. It also challenges your stability and balance since you are standing on one leg. You should use lighter weights than when just doing shoulder presses standing on both legs.

Pick up the dumbbells and hold them by your sides with your palms facing forward. Stand on your right leg, and flex both elbows, bringing the dumbbells closer to your upper arms (1). Then bring your elbows out to the sides so that your palms face forward and your forearms are straight up and down. Push the dumbbells straight up and slightly toward each other, straightening out your elbows into a shoulder press (2). Repeat on the left leg.

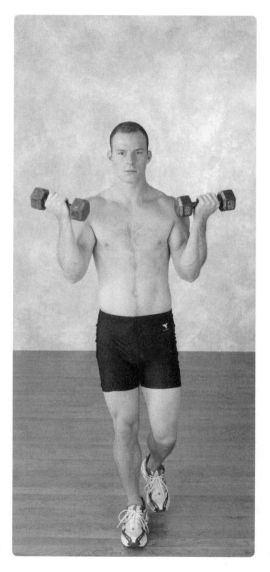

1

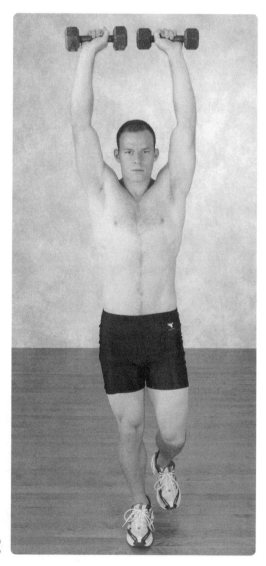

2

Standing Single-Arm Shoulder Press With Tubing

This exercise targets your deltoids and triceps. Stand on the tubing with both feet, about halfway between the center and the left grip. Hold the other grip with your right hand. Bring your right upper arm out to the side at shoulder height and bend your elbow to about 90 degrees, with your forearm pointing up (1). As you exhale, straighten out the arm at the elbow (2). Keep your wrist neutral the entire time, not allowing it to flex or extend as you do the movement. You can move your feet slightly to the left if you want to feel less resistance from the tubing or slightly to the right for more resistance. When you finish your repetitions, repeat on the opposite side.

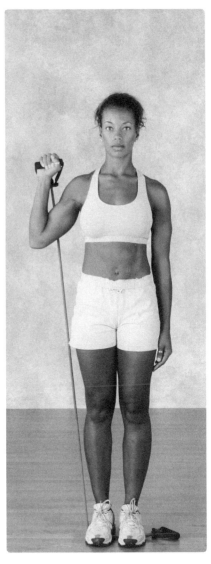
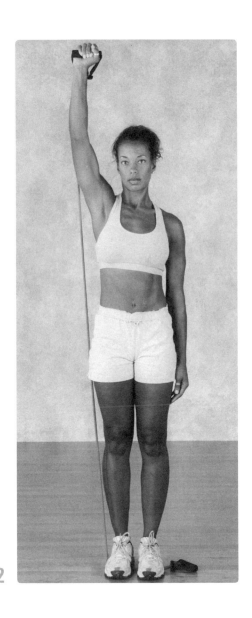

Standing Horizontal Row With Dumbbells

This targets your rhomboids, middle trapezius, posterior deltoids, and triceps. When you think about the names of exercises, it is important to remember that "horizontal" refers to the plane in which the movement occurs relative to your body, with the torso generally representing the "vertical" plane even if it happens not to be upright. When you do this horizontal row with dumbbells, you need to lean over so that you are working away from gravity—your arms are still moving "horizontally" relative to the position of your torso, even though they move vertically relative to gravity.

Holding a dumbbell in each hand, lean forward from your hips. Be sure to maintain the natural curve in your low back, and keep your knees soft and your abs strong. Let your arms hang straight down from your shoulders, with your knuckles facing the floor (1). As you exhale, pull your elbows out to the sides and up toward the ceiling (2). Pull your shoulder blades down and back at the same time. You should be looking at the floor to keep your neck neutral.

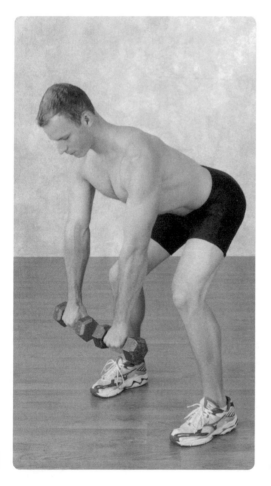
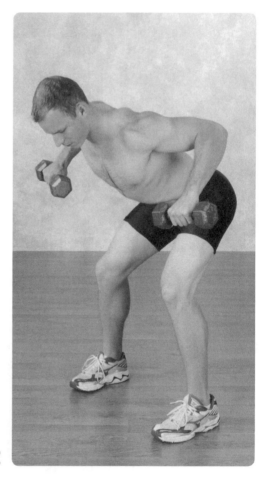

1　　　　2

Horizontal Row With Cable

This targets your upper middle back and posterior deltoids. Stand facing the cable, which should be coming from chest height. Use a double-handled attachment at the end of the cable and hold a grip in each hand. Stand with your right leg a little in front of your left. Let your arms straighten out in front of you parallel to the floor, allowing your shoulder blades to separate (1). You should be standing far enough away from the cable so that the weights do not touch as you get started. Exhale and pull your shoulder blades together as you pull your elbows back behind you (2).

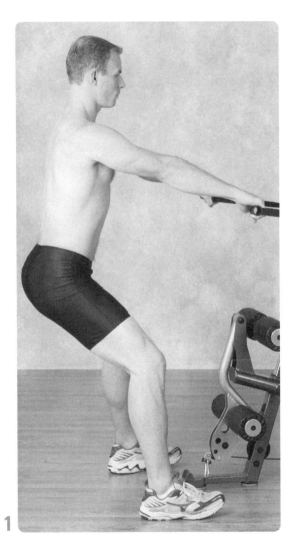

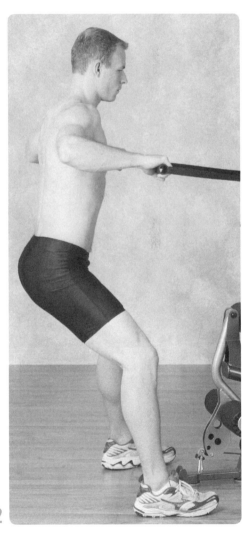

Standing Lateral Lunge With Single-Arm Horizontal Row and Tubing

This targets your rhomboids, middle trapezius, posterior deltoids, and triceps, as well as the muscles of your legs, especially the adductors. It's a great example of an exercise that combines an upper-body with a lower-body movement.

Attach the tubing around a stable object at about chest height so you can hold one grip in your right hand. Stand far enough away from the object to feel a little tension as you start the movement. Hold the tubing up so that your arm is pointing straight in front of you at about shoulder height (1). Step out to the right with your right leg, bending the right knee and pushing your hips back. At the same time, pull your right arm back, bending at the elbow and keeping it at shoulder height (2). Step back to the center, allowing your right arm to straighten out again. When you finish your repetitions, repeat on the opposite side.

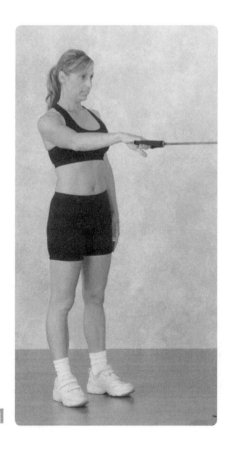

1

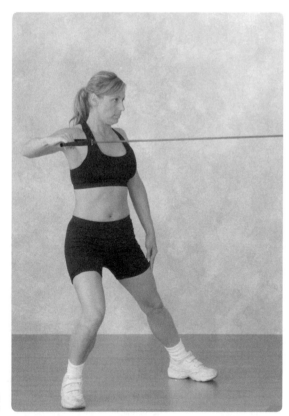

2

Standing Lateral Lunge With Single-Arm Horizontal Row and Cable

Like the previous exercise, this targets your rhomboids, middle trapezius, posterior deltoids, and triceps, as well as the muscles of your legs, especially the adductors. It's another great example of combining an upper-body with a lower-body movement.

Set the cable so it is at about shoulder height and hold the grip in your right hand. Stand far enough away from the cable so you feel a little tension as you start the movement. Hold the cable up, stretching your arm out in front of you at about shoulder height (1). Step out to the right with your right leg, bending the right knee and pushing your hips back. At the same time, pull your right arm back, bending at the elbow and keeping it at shoulder height (2). Step back to the center, allowing your right arm to straighten out in front of you once more. When you finish your repetitions, repeat on the opposite side.

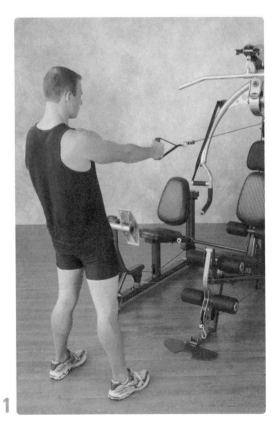

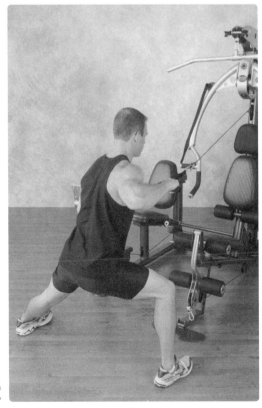

Horizontal Row on Machine

This targets your posterior deltoids, rhomboids, and middle trapezius. Adjust the seat height so that when you hold the horizontal handles your arms are at or just below shoulder height. Grip the handles with palms facing down and thumbs facing each other (1). As you exhale, pull your elbows back, pulling your shoulder blades down and back at the same time (2). You should wind up with your elbows bent to about 90 degrees.

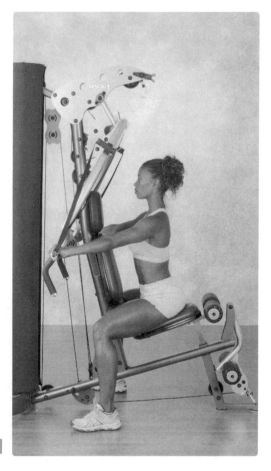

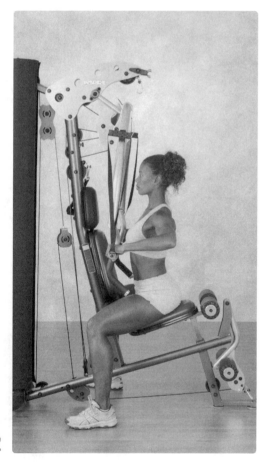

1

2

Reach, Roll, and Lift

I discussed this exercise in chapter 4, explaining its benefits for people who have poor posture, with their shoulders rounded forward. It is also good to do it if your upper trapezius muscle tends to feel tight. The main purpose of the exercise is to get your lower trapezius to fire, which in turn helps relax the upper trapezius.

Kneel on the floor, then sit back with your butt resting on your heels. Let your upper body relax so that your head rests on the floor with your arms stretched forward next to it, palms on the floor. In yoga practice, this position is known as the child's pose. Keeping your arms straight at the elbows, slide them farther forward on the floor, moving from your shoulder girdle. It should feel like you are shrugging your shoulders. This is the "reach" part of the exercise (1). Move your arms forward and back three times. Then reach again, hold the outstretched position, and externally rotate your whole arm. This involves turning your thumbs up toward the ceiling and out to the sides, but try to start the motion all the way back from your shoulders so that both of your entire arms are turning. This is the "roll" part. Do this sequence three times: reach, roll the arms, unroll them, and then pull them back to the starting position. After the third repetition, do it once more and stay in the reached and rolled position, then lift your arms up and down 10 times (2). Unroll your arms and pull them back.

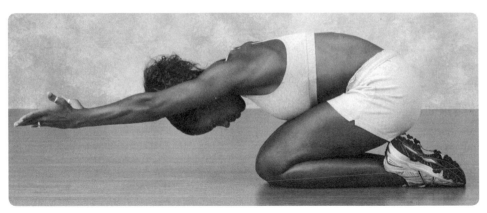

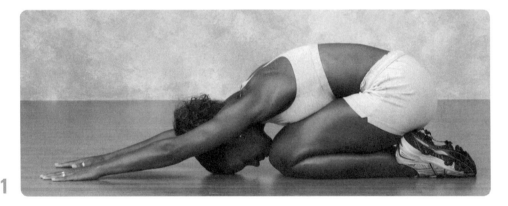

11

Core

Your core is composed of the muscles that connect your pelvis to your rib cage. The ultimate goal of strengthening the core muscles that make up your midriff is to stabilize your spine. This will make you stronger from the inside out, helping to transfer forces both up and down and support the entire body. The most important core stability muscles from deep to superficial are the pelvic floor, transverse abdominis, multifidus (very small muscles in between the vertebrae of your spine), internal and external obliques, and rectus abdominis. Working the rectus abdominis by doing crunches has gotten the most attention through the years, because many of our exercise programs come to us from bodybuilders, who isolate specific muscles in order to get them bigger. We now know, though, that the deeper core muscles you cannot see on the surface are very important as well.

To properly perform core exercises, you should first become familiar with the sensation of engaging the deep muscles in your core. Lie on your back with your knees bent and your feet flat on the floor, legs hip-width apart. Find your neutral spine, or the natural curve of your low back, by deliberately flattening your low back to the floor and then moving your pelvis in the opposite direction, arching your low back. Find the in-between point that feels normal to you and try to maintain that. Put your hands on your belly, one on each side of your navel. Inhale through your nose. You should feel your belly rise, without feeling any tension at your neck. You should not see or feel your chest rising. Forcefully exhale through your mouth. Now you should feel your navel being pulled in gently. You should be able to do this without any change in the curve of your low back—that is, maintaining a neutral spine. Then as you maintain normal breathing, try to keep your navel pulled in slightly as your belly rises and falls. This simple posture is essential to get your core muscles firing in the proper sequence to help stabilize your spine. Even though maintaining this integrity may be challenging, it is crucial for the effectiveness of the exercise and for your safety.

Some movements in core exercises, such as flexing and rotating, target specific muscles. You can also do core exercises in which the goal is to keep your trunk perfectly still, with no movement at your spine. These are often referred to as stabilizing exercises. In these exercises, the muscles in and around your core are isometrically contracted, that is, contracted without actually producing movement. As you perform them, you should feel your navel gently pulled in, and your hip bones should remain still. When you find that you can no longer maintain this stillness, you should either stop the exercise or make it easier. The purpose of stabilizing exercises is to make the internal firing mechanism more efficient so that you don't have to stress other areas of your body unnecessarily during your workout and to help you sustain stability for longer periods of time. Being able to stabilize your body properly also allows you to lift more weight, which will improve the results of your morning strength training. This chapter contains both exercises that target specific muscles and exercises for stability.

Toe Tap

This is a stabilizing exercise. Lie on your back with your knees bent, feet on the floor about hip-width apart. Place your hands on your hip bones where they protrude in two points above your thighs, below and to the sides of your navel, so you can feel whether you are able to keep them still as you do the exercise. Exhale, pulling your abdominal muscles in gently. Maintain that position as you continue breathing (1). Lift your left foot one inch (about two and a half centimeters) off the floor (2), keeping your leg bent, then lower it back to the floor. You should not feel your hip bones shifting. If you do, keep working on this first step before you continue. Lift your right foot one inch (about two and a half centimeters) off the floor, then lower it. Continue alternating for up to a total of 15 repetitions on each side. You can tell if your core muscles get fatigued before then by noticing what else is going on in your body. For example, if you start feeling tension in your neck or you see that your belly is popping up, you should stop the exercise and rest.

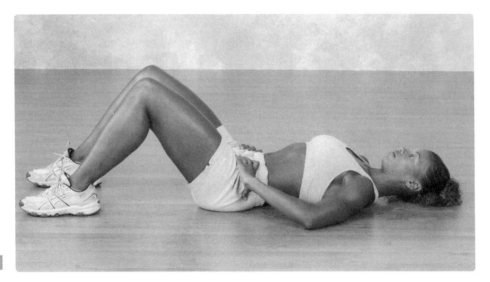

1

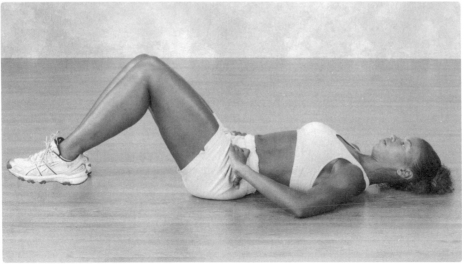

2

Toe Tap With Longer Leg

This stabilizing exercise is a more difficult variation of the toe-tap exercise described previously. Lie on your back with your knees bent, feet on the floor about hip-width apart. Place your hands on your hip bones where they protrude in two points above your thighs, below and to the sides of your navel, so you can feel whether you are able to keep them still as you do the exercise (1).

Exhale, pulling your abdominal muscles in gently. Lift your right foot one inch (about two and a half centimeters) off the floor. With your foot in the air, straighten the leg, keeping your foot a few inches off the floor (2), then bend it back to the original angle and lower the foot back to the floor. The longer you make your leg, the harder it will be to stay still in your core and to keep your hip bones still. Switch to the left side, and continue alternating for up to a total of 15 repetitions on each side.

1

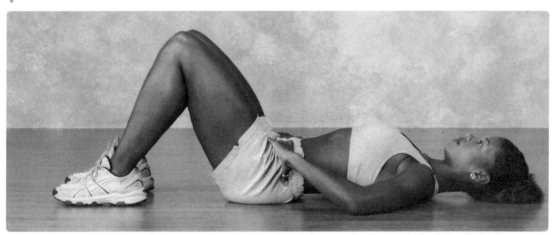

2

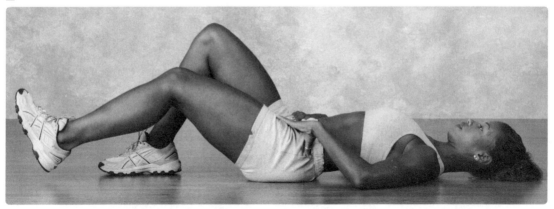

Toe Tap With Both Feet Up

This stabilizing exercise is more difficult than the previous two because both feet are starting up off the floor. Lie on your back and lift up first your right foot and then your left foot so that both feet are in the air, with your hips and knees bent to 90 degrees. This is your starting position (1). Pull your abdominal muscles in gently and maintain your neutral spine as you lower your right toes to the floor (2), tap gently, and lift back up to the starting position. Alternate legs for up to a total of 15 repetitions on each side. Again, you can make this more challenging by straightening your leg a little as you bring it to the floor.

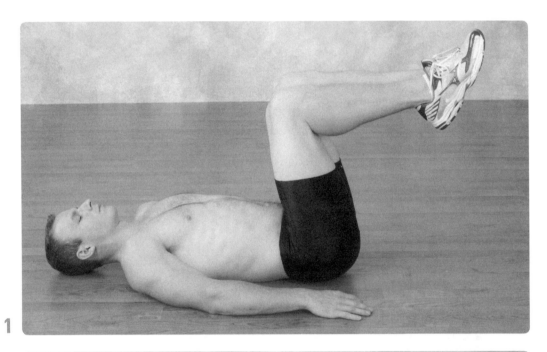

1

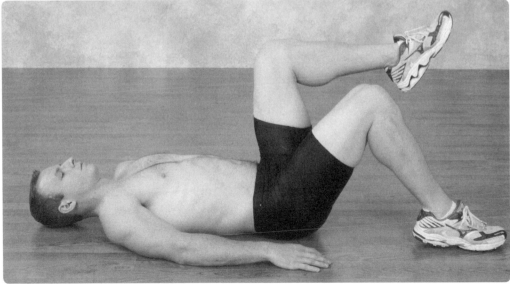

2

Reverse Chop With Cable

This is a strengthening exercise. Stand with your left side next to the cable; the cable should be coming from the bottom. Stand far enough away from the cable to feel some resistance before you start the exercise. Hold the grip with both hands. Squat and turn toward the cable, flexing at your spine, as if you were picking something up from outside your left foot (1). Then stand up, bringing your arms across the front of your body and up and out over your right shoulder (2). Keep your elbows relatively straight throughout the motion, and think about making a diagonal line across the front of your body.

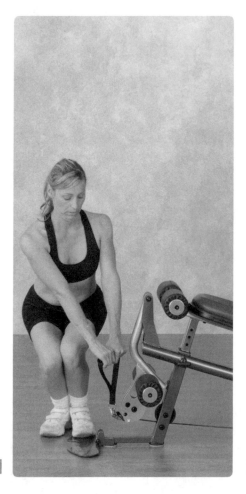

1

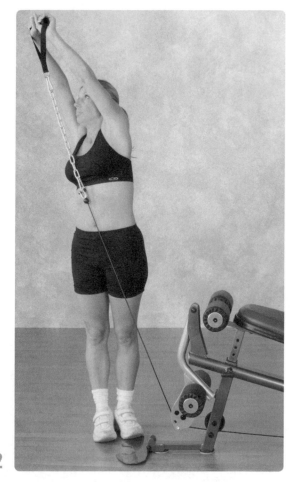

2

Opposite Arm/Leg Reach

This exercise is for core stability. It targets the muscles along your spine more than exercises that have you lying on your back can do. This is because of your position relative to gravity—unlike when you are lying on the floor, the muscles along your spine have to hold you up away from gravity. You will feel how challenging this exercise is if you try to keep your hip bones perfectly still the entire time.

Get on all fours, with your hands right under your shoulders and your knees right under your hips (1). Lift your right arm and your left leg at the same time. Face your palm to the floor, and keep your elbow straight but not locked out. Straighten out your left leg as you lift it so that your body is in a straight line, parallel to the floor (2). Your foot should be facing toward the floor, and your leg should be in line with your hips, not out to the side. Hold them in the lengthened position for three to five seconds, and then bring them back to the starting position. Switch sides.

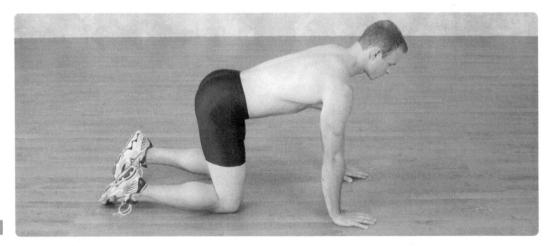

1

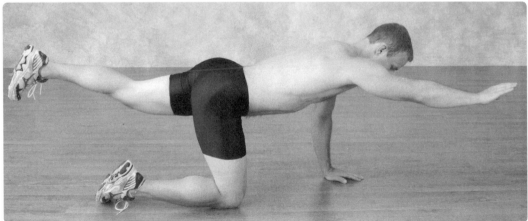

2

Prone Hold on Forearms

This exercise challenges your core stability and also your shoulder stability, since you are resting on your forearms. Lie facedown on the floor and then put your elbows under your shoulders so that your upper body is propped up on your forearms. Curl your toes under so that the balls of your feet are resting on the ground. Now, pull your abdominal muscles in and lift your hips up off the floor so your whole body is supported by your forearms and your toes. Your eyes should be facing the floor to keep your neck neutral. Your body should be in a straight line from your shoulders to your toes; make sure your butt isn't up in the air. Stop when you feel gentle shaking through your midsection. Try to work up to holding the position for 30 seconds. You can modify this exercise by keeping your knees on the floor.

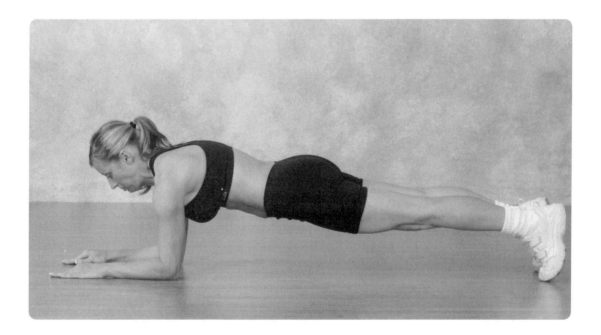

Prone Hold on Hands

This is essentially the same as the prone hold on forearms except that in this one your arms are straight. This is more challenging for your wrists and arms but easier on your core, since your upper body is a little farther away from the floor and your center of gravity is closer to your feet.

Start on your hands and knees with your hands directly under your shoulders and your elbows straight but not locked. While maintaining a neutral spine, straighten out one leg so that you get your toes on the floor. Then straighten out your other leg. Your legs should be hip-width apart. Your eyes should be facing the floor to keep your neck neutral. Your body should be in a straight line from your shoulders to your toes; make sure your butt isn't up in the air. Stop when you feel gentle shaking through your midsection. Try to work up to holding the position for 30 seconds. You can modify this exercise by keeping your knees on the floor.

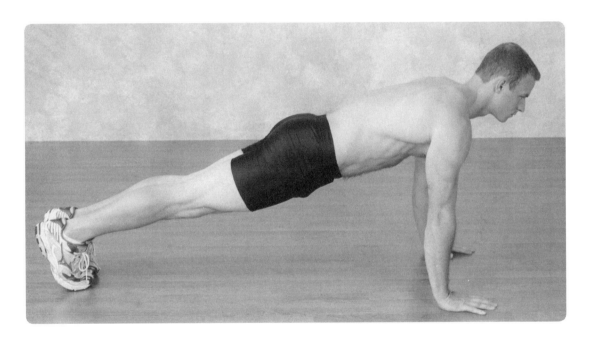

Lateral Hold on Forearm

This core stability exercise challenges your core as well as the lateral muscles along the side of your body. These muscles are your deltoids, lat muscle, quadratus lumborum (a deep core stabilizer that connects your pelvis to your spine and rib cage), and gluteus medius and minimus (the muscles of your outer hip).

Lie on your right side and place your right elbow directly under your right shoulder. Pull your abdominal muscles in and lift your hips up off the floor. Your body should form a straight line from your head to your feet. Hold for as long as you can, and work up to 30 seconds. Do the same on the left side. You can modify this exercise by keeping your knees on the floor.

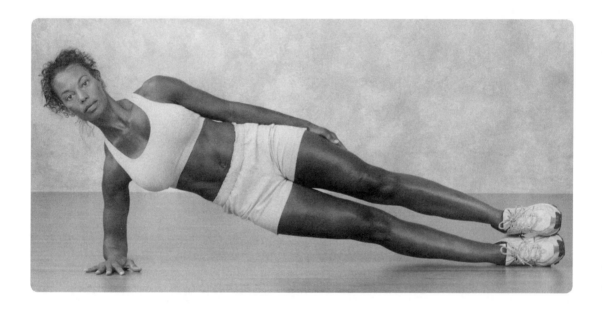

Lateral Hold With Straight Arm

Like the previous core stability exercise, this challenges your core as well as the lateral muscles along the side of your body. These muscles are your deltoids, lat muscle, quadratus lumborum (a deep core stabilizer that connects your pelvis to your spine and rib cage), and gluteus medius and minimus (the muscles of your outer hip). The main difference between doing this exercise with a straight arm and doing it on your forearm is that doing it with a straight arm challenges your arm strength and your wrist integrity, although in terms of holding yourself up against gravity this variation is actually easier.

Lie on your right side. Place your right hand directly under your right shoulder and straighten the arm so that your upper body and hips are lifted off the ground. Your body should form a straight line from your head to your feet. Pull your abdominal muscles in when you lift your hips up off the floor. Hold for as long as you can, and work up to 30 seconds. Do the same on your left side.

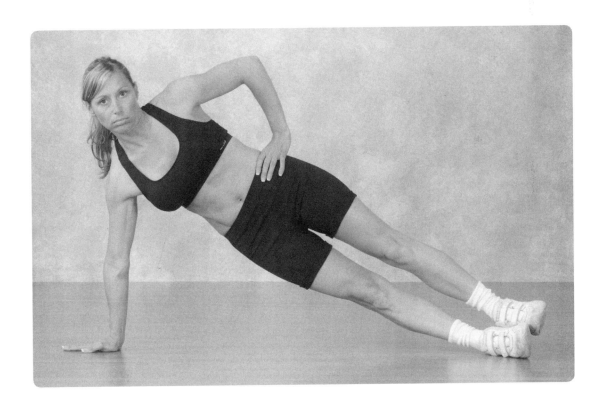

Hanging Leg Raise

This exercise challenges your entire core to stay still as you lift your legs, and the lifting makes you work your hip flexors. It is also a great way to strengthen the integrity of your shoulders, your forearms, and your grip. Hang from a bar, using an overhand grip and letting your arms stay straight (1). Pulling in your abs, lift your knees up as high as possible while maintaining a neutral spine (2), and bring them down again. Try to keep your upper body still as you lift and lower your knees.

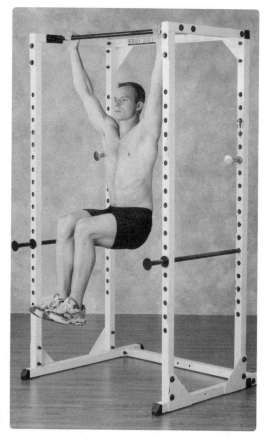

1

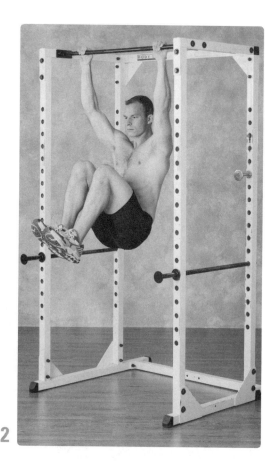

2

Seated Rotation With Dumbbell

This exercise targets the internal and external obliques, which help rotate your body from side to side. As you move at your spine during the exercise, you should still be thinking of that gentle core stability from the inside out, feeling that your navel is being held pulled in. Sit on the floor with your feet out in front of you and your knees bent. Sit up tall, keeping your abs pulled in, your spine neutral, and your chest up. Hold a dumbbell out in front of you with both hands, keeping your arms straight but not locked (1). The dumbbell should be straight up and down. Turn your body from side to side (2), making sure that you move your whole trunk and not just your arms.

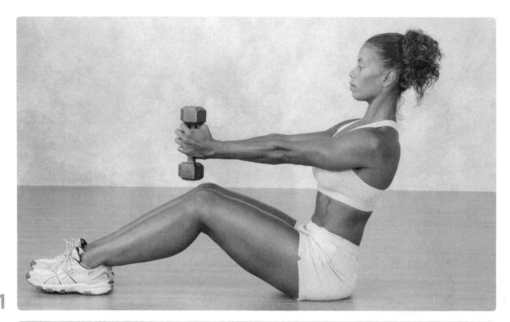

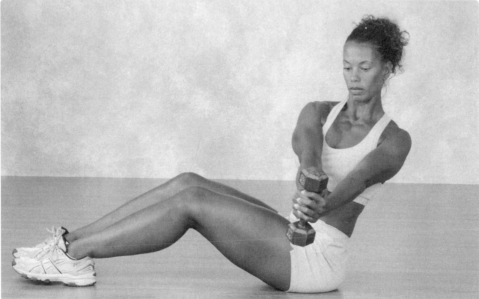

Standing Rotation With Tubing

This exercise targets your internal and external obliques, along with your deep stabilizers. Wrap a piece of tubing around a sturdy object so that it is at about the height of your midsection. Stand with the left side of your body facing the tubing. Hold the tubing with both hands out in front of your body with your elbows straight but not locked (1). Turn your body to the right, moving at your spine and your hips, keeping your arms in front of your upper body in the same relative position as when you started (2). You should feel that your left foot wants to come up off the floor as you rotate. When you are finished with your set, turn around so the right side of your body is facing the tubing, and rotate to the left.

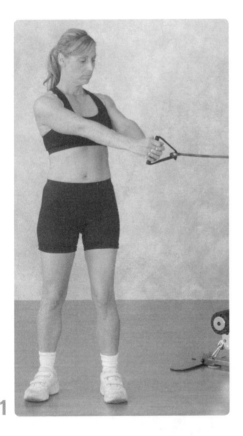

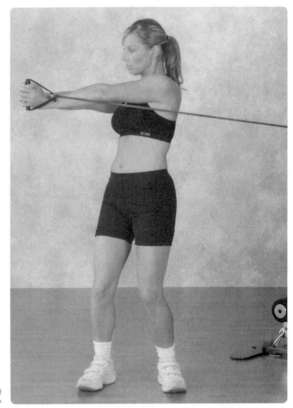

Standing Rotation With Cable

This exercise targets your internal and external obliques, along with your deep stabilizers. Set the cable at about the height of your midsection. Stand with the left side of your body facing the cable. Hold the grip with both hands out in front of your body, keeping your elbows straight but not locked (1). Turn your body to the right, moving at your spine and your hips, keeping your arms positioned directly in front of you as you move (2). You should feel that your left foot wants to come up off the floor as you rotate. When you are finished with your set, turn around so the right side of your body is facing the cable, and rotate to the left.

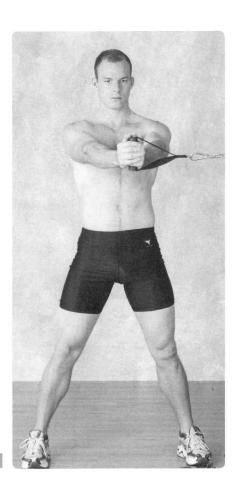
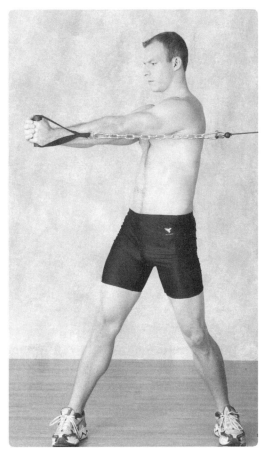

1

2

Oblique Crunch

This targets your rectus abdominis and your internal and external obliques. Lie down on your back, with your knees bent and your feet off the floor. You should have 90-degree angles at your hips and knees. Interlace your hands behind your head (1). Inhale, and then as you exhale, curl up and bring your right shoulder toward your left hip (2). Alternate sides.

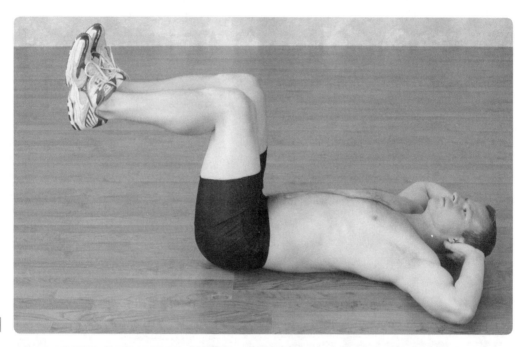

1

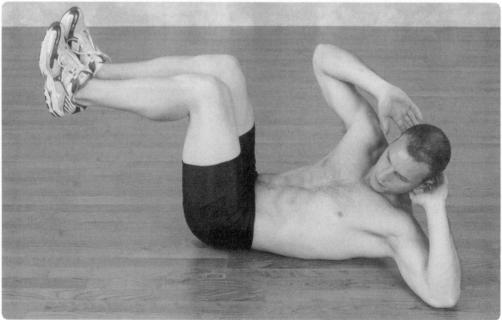

2

Reverse Crunch

This exercise targets your rectus abdominis. The movement begins at your pelvis, which is where this muscle group starts. Lie on your back with your hips and knees both bent at 90-degree angles. Keep your arms out to the sides (1). Exhale, pull your abs in and flatten out your low back as you curl your spine from the bottom side (2). Keep your thighs vertical; the angle at your hips should not change. This is the same action as a traditional crunch, except that you are flexing your spine from the bottom side as opposed to the top side. You should not feel any stress in your neck or upper body. The stronger you get, the more you will be able to curl your butt up off the floor.

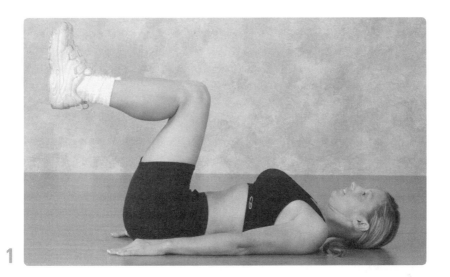

1

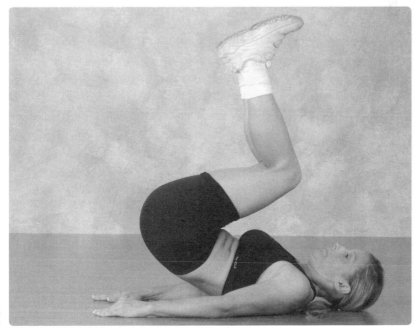

2

Supine Rotation

This exercise targets the internal and external obliques and the deep stabilizing muscles of the core. Lie on your back with both your hips and knees bent at 90-degree angles so that your feet are up in the air. Spread your arms out to the side, forming a letter T with your body (1). Let your legs fall slowly to the left, stopping just before they reach the ground, using your abs to control the movement (2). Inhale, then exhale as you bring your legs back to the center and over to the right side. Try to push into your arms as little as possible. You can increase the difficulty of the exercise by straightening your legs a little more so that your lower legs are more vertical.

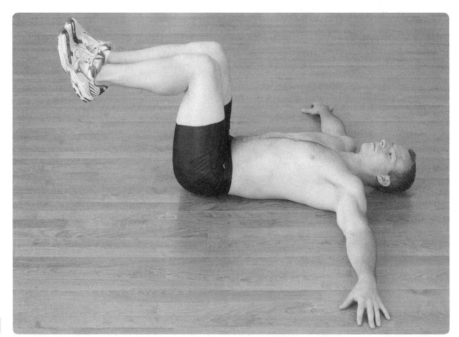

1

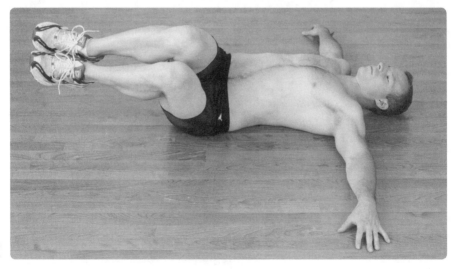

2

Back Extension

This exercise targets the extensor muscles along your spine. You will also use your glutes to help keep still as you lift your upper body off the ground. Lie facedown on the floor with your arms resting down by your sides, palms turned up (1). Lift your upper body up off the floor as high as you can without straining. At the same time, pull your shoulders down and back and look toward the floor to keep your neck neutral (2). Hold for five seconds, and then lower your upper body to the floor. You can increase the difficulty by lifting your legs at the same time as your upper body.

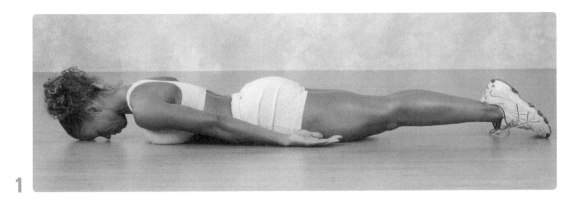

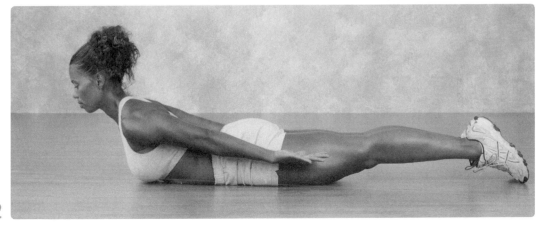

Crunch on Stability Ball

This exercise targets your rectus abdominis, initiating the movement from the top (the insertion) of the muscle group. It also challenges the muscles around your hips to keep you still on the ball as you do the exercise. Sit on the ball and then walk forward, lying back onto it. The size of the ball should be such that you get a feeling of extension, or opening up, in the front of your body as you lie down. Start the exercise with the ball at your low back. Place your hands behind your head, and keep your neck relaxed throughout the exercise (1). Exhale as you curl up, coming up as high as you can without straining (2). You can make this more challenging by straightening out one or both arms.

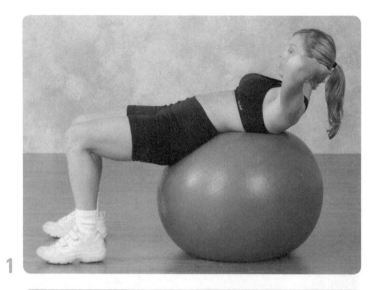

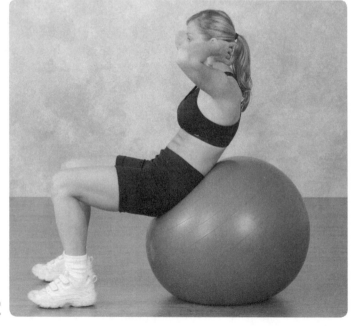

Crunch on Stability Ball With Medicine Ball

This exercise targets your rectus abdominis, initiating the movement from the top (the insertion) of the muscle group. It also challenges the muscles around your hips to stay still on the ball as you do the exercise. Holding a medicine ball adds extra resistance. The farther away from your body you hold the medicine ball, the harder the exercise becomes.

Sit on the stability ball and then walk forward as you lie back on it. The size of the ball should be such that you get a feeling of extension, or opening up, in the front as you lie down. Start with the ball at your low back. Hold the medicine ball in your hands, and keep your neck relaxed (1). You can start the exercise with the medicine ball at your chest, then progress by holding the medicine ball at your forehead or over your head as you do the exercise. Exhale as you curl up, coming up as high as you can without straining (2).

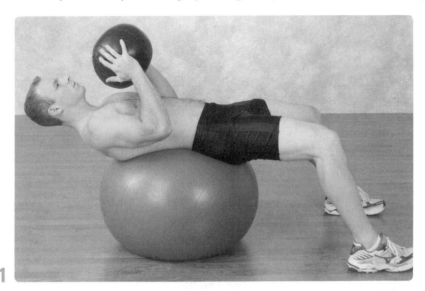

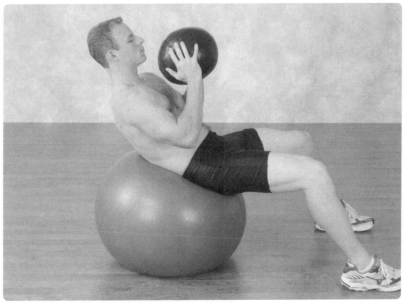

Prone Hold on Stability Ball

This targets your entire core, which has to work against gravity to stabilize you on the ball. It also challenges your shoulder girdle and shoulder joints. Kneel facing the stability ball with your body close to it, and place your forearms on top of it and your elbows directly under your shoulders (1). Straighten your knees and rise onto your toes (2). Hold the position, or move your arms in small circles, moving the stability ball several times in each direction.

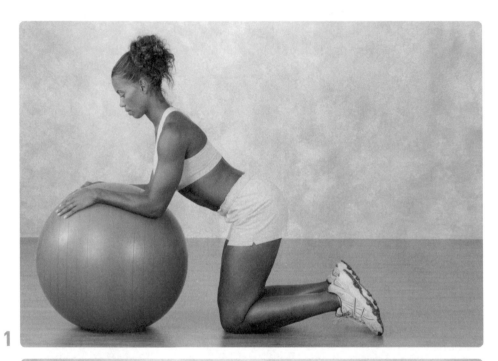

1

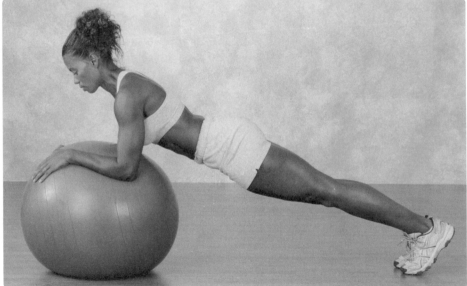

2

Crab Walk

This targets your entire core, plus your upper body, since your arms are helping to hold you up against gravity. Get on the floor as if beginning a push-up, putting your hands below your shoulders with your arms straight and rising onto your toes (1). Move to the right, lifting up your arms and legs to move (2). "Walk" about five to ten steps to the right and then back to the left. Try to keep your hips down, with your body forming a straight line. You can make it more challenging by placing your hands farther forward on the floor instead of directly under your shoulders.

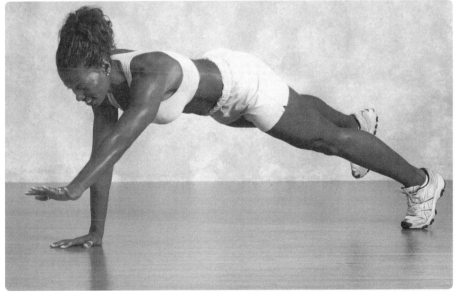

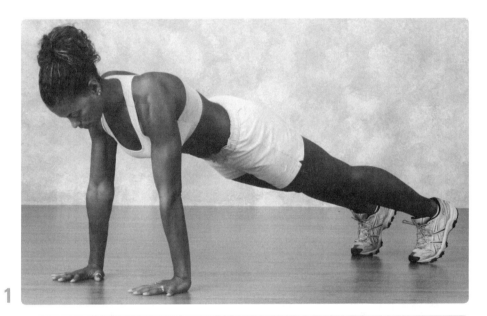

Standing Chop With Cable

This exercise targets all of your core muscles. Set the cable above shoulder height. Stand with the left side of your body facing the cable. Hold the grip with both hands. Turn toward the left, keeping your arms straight (1). Exhale as you pull the cable toward your right hip, turning your upper body as you pull (2).

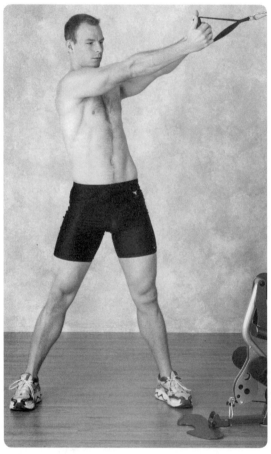

1

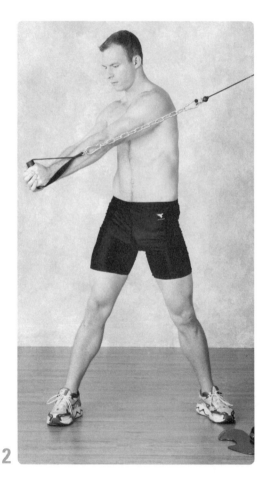

2

12

Lower Body

|||||||||||||||||||||||||||||||||||||||||||||||||||||||||||||||||||||||||||||||||||||||||||||||||||||||||||||||||||||||||||||||||||||||||||||

The lower-body exercises use muscles that work around the hip, knee, and ankle joints.

• **Hip.** Your hip joint is basically where your femur, or thigh bone, connects to your acetabulum, which is a deep socket in your pelvis. The movements at your hip include flexion, bringing your thigh and torso closer together in the front, and extension, which is bringing them farther apart, essentially moving your leg behind the line of your body. Abduction is bringing your leg out to the side, away from the midline of your body, and adduction is bringing it toward the midline. External hip rotation is turning your entire leg out, and internal rotation is turning your entire leg in.

Hip flexion is produced by the iliopsoas mucle group, as well as the rectus femoris, one of the quadriceps muscles. Hip extension is done with your gluteus maximus and your hamstrings: biceps femoris, semitendinosus, and semimembranosus. The gluteus medius and minimus produce hip abduction, and the pectineus; adductor brevis, longus, and magnus; and the gracilis are in the group called the adductors. External rotation is caused by the piriformis, the gemellus superior and inferior, the obturator internus and externus, and the quadratus femoris. Internal rotation is done by several muscles including the adductors and the gluteus medius and minimus.

The muscles around your hip move your leg in the directions described, as well as stabilize your sacroiliac (SI) joint when working together as in a squat or a lunge. Your SI joint is where your sacrum, the triangle bone at the bottom of your spine, meets your pelvis at both sides, right in between your glute muscles in the back.

• **Knee.** The knee joint is where the femur, or thigh bone, meets the tibia from below, and the patella, or knee cap, sits in between. The movements at the knee are flexion and extension. Knee flexion is done by the hamstrings. Knee extension is done by the quadriceps: the rectus femoris, vastus lateralis, vastus medialis, and vastus intermedius.

• **Ankle.** The ankle joint is where the tibia and the fibula meet the calcaneus, or heel bone. The movements at this joint are dorsiflexion, decreasing the angle between your shin and your foot, and plantarflexion, increasing the angle. There is also inversion and eversion. Inversion means your foot lifts up on the inside, putting your weight on the outside edge, and eversion is the opposite. Pronation and supination, which are movements along all three planes at once, occur at the subtalar joint where the foot and ankle meet. This is discussed in chapter 4. Basically, pronation is when your arch collapses, and your whole lower leg rotates in. Supination is when your arch lifts up, and your whole lower leg rotates out.

The major moves of the ankle are dorsiflexion from your tibialis anterior and plantarflexion, which is produced by the calf muscles gastrocnemius and soleus, as well as the tibialis posterior. Inversion, eversion, supination, and pronation are very integrated movements, meaning that many muscles contribute to these movements.

The exercises in this book address all of the movements possible for the lower body. Some of these lower-body exercises target particular muscle groups, while others work the entire lower body at once. The first exercises listed in this chapter are those that work more than one muscle group at a time—various kinds of squats and lunges; a deadlift using a barbell; and bridges using a stability ball and just your body. Next come band walking and heel raises, which target specific muscle groups. Finally, there are leg presses (which work your whole lower body) and leg extension (which targets the quadriceps)—both of these types of exercises are great ways to work your lower body using traditional machines at a gym.

Three major categories of lower-body exercises are squats, lunges, and bridges.

• **Squats.** A squat is an example of a functional exercise in that it simulates everyday movement. In order to sit down onto a chair, you have to perform some sort of squat! Many people believe, wrongly, that doing a squat exercise will hurt their knees. This misconception has come about because people often do squats incorrectly, failing to push their hips back as they bend their knees. This puts undue pressure on the knees and prevents your body from absorbing the forces in the way it is designed to do. The best way to do a squat is to keep in mind that you want to move three joints—your ankle, your knee, and your hip—at the same time. The different parts of your body are meant to work in unison, as a chain, dissipating the force that the ground exerts onto your body. A squat works your whole lower body all at one time. When you perform squats in your workouts, go down until your thighs are about parallel to the floor, or stop before then if you lose your neutral spine or your upper body tilts forward so much that you're no longer more or less upright.

• **Lunges.** Like a squat, a lunge works your whole lower body at the same time. Unlike a squat, however, a lunge requires your legs to move in opposite directions at your hips, with your core muscles stabilizing your pelvis as you do so. Incorporating lunges into your workouts will increase your fitness and will help you do everyday activities such as walking up and down the stairs, stepping toward and reaching for something on the floor, and even playing sports like tennis. To do a basic lunge, start by standing with your feet hip-width apart. Take a step back with your right leg, about 2 to 3 feet (.6 to 1 meter). Keeping your spine neutral, bend both knees to 90 degrees at the same time. If your back knee does not get to 90 degrees, you need to take a longer step. Your front heel should stay on the floor as you lunge, and the back heel needs to come up off the floor.

• **Bridges.** A bridge is a great exercise to help stabilize your sacroiliac (SI) joint, as well as to strengthen your glutes and hamstrings. You can do many different types of bridges as you will soon see! To do a bridge, lie face up on the floor, legs hip-width apart, with your knees bent to about 90 degrees and your feet on the floor. Maintaining a neutral spine, lift up your hips as you exhale, and inhale as you lower your hips back to the floor. You can do bridges with one or two legs, and you can increase the challenge by putting your upper or lower body on a stability ball.

Free-Standing Squat With Dumbbells

This targets your whole lower body. Stand with your feet hip- to shoulder-width apart and your feet pointing forward (not turned out). Hold one dumbbell in each hand (1). Inhale as you flex your ankles, knees, and hips at the same time, going down toward the floor (2). You should feel your shins moving forward slightly into ankle dorsiflexion and your butt going back at the same time as you flex your hips. When you reach the point where your thighs are about parallel to the floor, or when you are about to lose your neutral spine, exhale and stand back up again.

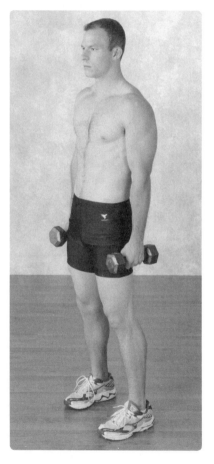

1

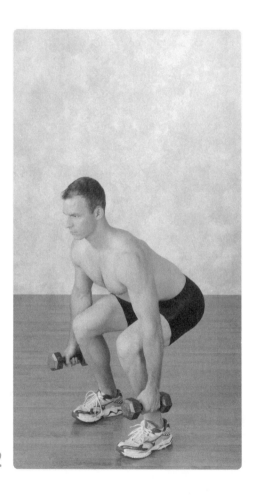

2

Squat With Barbell

This exercise works your entire lower body. Because you are holding the bar on your upper trapezius and need to stabilize the bar on your body as you do the exercise, it also challenges your core. Since you are bearing the weight on your upper body but moving it with your entire lower body, you can handle a relatively heavy weight—certainly more than you could by just holding a dumbbell in each hand. For this reason, you may also notice your heart rate increasing if you pick a weight that feels challenging.

Set up the barbell on the squat rack so that it is slightly lower than your upper trapezius muscles (or slightly lower than your shoulders). It should be at a height where you will have to squat down slightly in order to get it behind your head, on your upper traps. Before you begin the exercise, put the safety mechanism in place on the squat rack. The safety mechanism should be set at a height so that if you had to stop the exercise, you could easily rest the barbell on the safety pieces and get out from underneath the bar. Also be sure to use the safety collars on the weights on the outside of the bar to prevent them from sliding off the ends.

Stand facing a mirror, with the bar on your upper traps. With an overhand grip, grasp the bar on each side with your hands about 4 inches (10 centimeters) more than shoulder-width apart, knuckles facing forward. Engage your core, stand up to lift the bar off the brackets, and step back a step or two in order to begin. Stand with your feet between hip- and shoulder-width apart, toes pointing forward (1). Inhale as you flex your ankles, knees, and hips at the same time, going down toward the floor (2). When you get to where your thighs are about parallel to the floor, or just before you lose your neutral spine, exhale and stand back up again. When you are finished with your set, walk forward to put the bar on the brackets and squat down slightly so you can step back away from the bar.

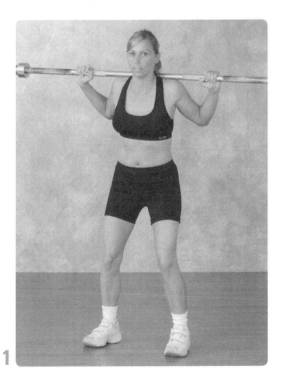
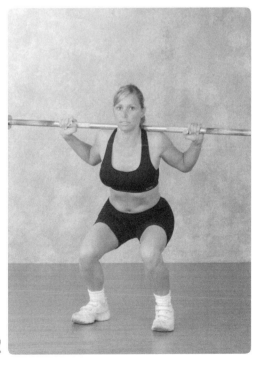

1

2

Single-Leg Squat

This works your entire leg at once. Since you are only using one leg to perform the movement, it can be quite challenging in terms of stabilization—you might notice that your knee wants to cave in as you do it. It's helpful to look at yourself in a mirror while you do single-leg squats and only go as deep as you can without your knee collapsing in.

Stand with your feet right next to each other, pointing straight ahead. Lift your left foot up off the ground and hold it next to the right one, keeping it close to the right foot but not pushing into it (1). Put your hands on your hips and flex at your right ankle, knee, and hip at the same time (2). You should think of pushing your hips back as you move toward the floor. Make sure your right knee stays in line with the foot and does not cave in as you bend. Go down until your right thigh is about parallel to the floor or until your leg starts collapsing in at the foot or knee. When you finish the repetitions on your right leg, switch sides.

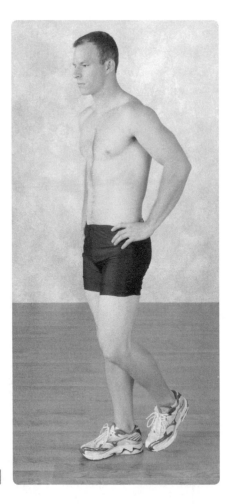

1

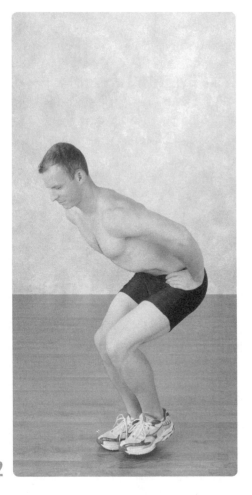

2

Single-Leg Squat With Opposite-Arm Reach

This exercise helps develop the balance of your entire body, since you are standing on one leg and then moving the opposite arm along different angles all around your body. The range of motion of your single-leg squat in this variation might be a little less than if you were just doing the squat by itself, since integrating a balance challenge into the exercise makes it more difficult.

Stand with your feet right next to each other and pointing straight ahead. Lift your left foot up and hold it next to the right one, keeping it close to the right foot but not pushing into it. Put your right hand on your right hip, and keep your left arm by your side (1). Flex at your right ankle, knee, and hip all at once; think of pushing your hips back as you move toward the floor. At the same time, reach across your body at waist height with your left arm. The next time you squat, reach your left arm a little higher across your body, at shoulder level (2). On the third squat, reach low across your body, toward your right foot. Continue alternating medium, high, and low reaches. Each time, squat down until your right thigh is about parallel to the floor, until your leg starts collapsing in at the foot or knee, or until you cannot maintain your balance and you need to keep putting your left foot down on the floor. Make sure your right knee stays in line with the foot and does not cave in as you bend. When you have finished your repetitions, switch sides.

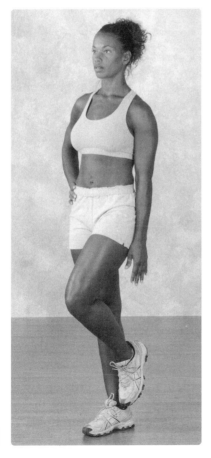
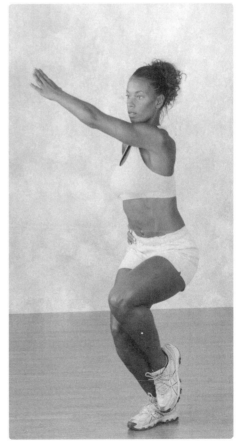

1

2

Squat Jump

This exercise works all the parts of your lower body together and derives much of its challenge from the jumping. The impact of jumping is very beneficial for your bone density. It also improves the ability of your joints and the proprioceptors around your joints to absorb force and react to changes of position as you exercise, go about your everyday life, or participate in sports. It is, however, extremely important to progress safely when incorporating jumping movements into your program. Think of a jump-rope exercise—it creates a very low level of impact, since you do not bend down very deep at all when you land. This is precisely how you should start your squat jumps.

To begin, stand in a squat position with your feet pointing straight ahead, between hip- and shoulder-width apart. Put your hands on your hips, squat down slightly toward the floor (1), and then jump up with your entire body (2) and land softly, bending at the knees, ankles, and hips. You should observe that your knees are not collapsing in a lot as you land. If your knees do cave in, include more of the single-leg squats in your workouts to develop the strength of each leg. You should also include the band walking exercise described later in this chapter. Your landings should be relatively quiet, which is a sign that your body is absorbing the force well and not putting too much strain on your joints.

If you are able to do one squat jump and hold your position for two or three seconds after landing without collapsing or losing your balance, then you can progress to doing three to five repetitions in a row. Once you can do more than five repetitions in a row with good form, you can try to do the squat jumps a tiny bit deeper, but again, do only three to five at a time. This is an important principle of safe progression—when you increase the difficulty of the exercise by making the range of motion greater, you should reduce the number of repetitions until you can do the deeper squats in good form; then you can continue the progressions. You can do up to eight repetitions, but be aware that the more you do, the harder it is to do them very deeply.

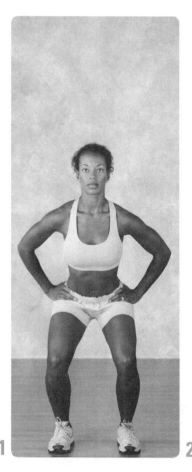
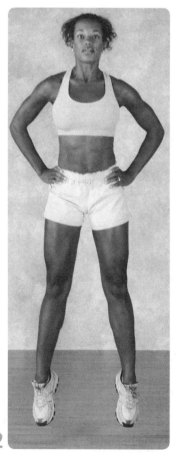

1 2

Stationary Lunge With Dumbbells

Stand with your feet hip-width apart, holding the dumbbells at your sides. Step forward about two feet (.6 meter) with your left foot (1). The length of your stride is correct when your knees are at right angles as you bend them. Bend both knees, stopping when your left thigh is parallel to the floor (2). Keeping your upper body still and tall, move up and down without losing this starting position. Your right heel will come up off the floor as you lower your body, but your left heel in front should stay on the floor. Switch sides after you finish your repetitions.

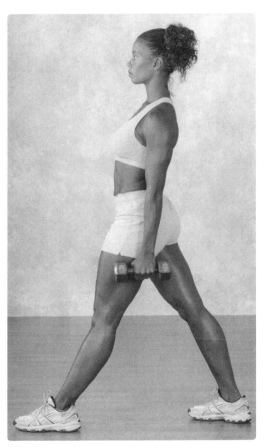

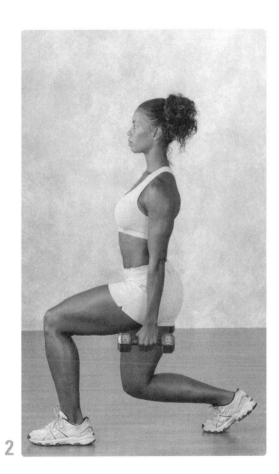

Reverse Lunge With Dumbbells

This exercise works on the whole lower body at once. Taking a step backward means that you challenge your proprioception (your awareness of where your body is in space) more than when doing a forward lunge. Stand with your feet hip-width apart, holding the dumbbells at your sides. Step backward about two feet (.6 meter) with your left foot (1). The length of your stride is correct when your knees are at right angles as you bend them. Bend both knees toward the floor, stopping when your right thigh is parallel to the floor (2). Your right heel should stay on the floor as you lower your body. Keeping your upper body still and tall, step forward with your left leg to the starting position and repeat. When you have finished your repetitions, switch sides.

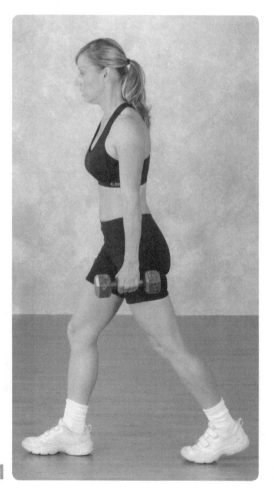
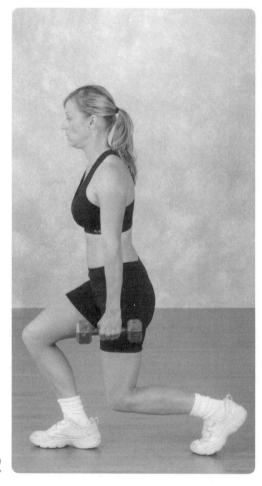

1 2

Walking Lunge With Dumbbells

This works your whole lower body at once. The walking adds an extra element of difficulty to this lunge. Stand with your feet hip-width apart, holding the dumbbells at your sides. Step forward about two feet (.6 meter) with your right foot. The length of your stride is correct when your knees are at right angles as you bend them. Bend both knees toward the floor, stopping when your right thigh is parallel to the floor (1). Keeping your upper body still and tall, push down with your right leg, coming up from the lunge (2), and bring your left leg forward to meet the right to where you are again standing on both feet. Now, start the next lunge by stepping forward with your left leg. As you get better at this exercise, you will be able to "walk" without having to rest in between steps to catch your breath or your balance.

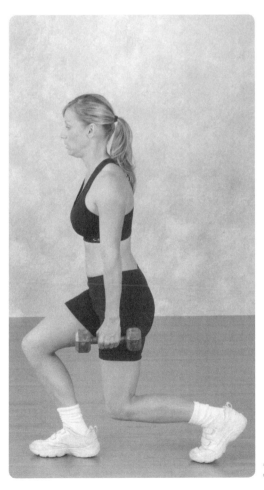

1

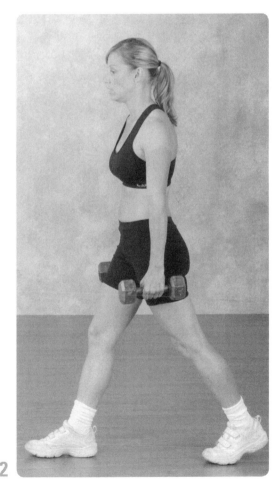

2

Walking Lunge With Rotation and Medicine Ball

This exercise is more integrated; the lunge works your whole lower body and the rotation with a medicine ball works your core. It's a very functional exercise, since in everyday life we often need to move our upper and lower bodies in different directions at the same time. Incorporating rotation into your routine is very good for stabilizing your spine, helping to keep your low back healthy. Start this exercise with a ball that is approximately 5 percent of your body weight. For example, if you weigh 130 pounds (about 60 kilograms), start with a medicine ball that weighs about 7 pounds (about 3 kilograms) and progress from there.

Stand with your feet hip-width apart, holding the medicine ball in front of your body at about waist height. Step forward about two feet (.6 meter) with your right foot. The length of your stride is correct when your knees are at right angles as you bend them (1). As you step with your right leg, rotate your upper body to the right. Make sure your entire upper body is rotating instead of just your arms moving from side to side. Bend both knees toward the floor, stopping when your right thigh is parallel to the floor (1). Keeping your upper body still and tall, push down with your right leg, coming up from the lunge, and bring your left leg forward to meet the right, standing on both feet. Now, start the next step with your left leg (2). As you step forward with your left leg into the lunge, rotate your entire upper body to the left. As you get better at this exercise, you will be able to walk without having to rest in between steps to catch your breath or your balance.

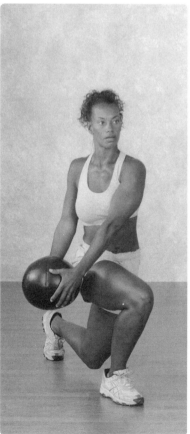

1

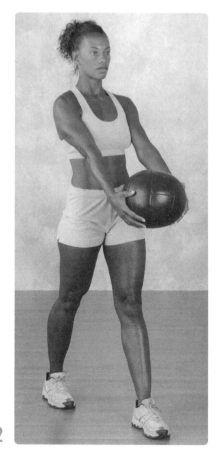

2

Lateral Lunge With Dumbbells

This works your whole lower body at the same time, with particular emphasis on your adductors, or inner thighs, which lengthen as you step to the opposite side. Traditional exercise programs have us moving forward and backward too much; it's important to include some lateral movement in your program, too.

Stand with your feet pointing straight ahead, hip-width apart, and hold a dumbbell in each hand (1). Step about three feet (just a bit under a meter) to the right with your right leg. Bend your right knee, pushing your hips back and keeping your left leg straight. Lean over your right thigh with one dumbbell on either side of your right leg (2). Raise your upper body again and return to the starting position. Repeat to the left side and continue alternating. A good way to think about this exercise is to pretend you are standing in the middle of a clock. Imagine that you're stepping to 3 o'clock when you lunge to the right, and imagine that you're stepping to 9 o'clock when you lunge to the left.

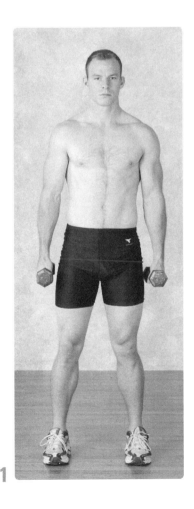

1

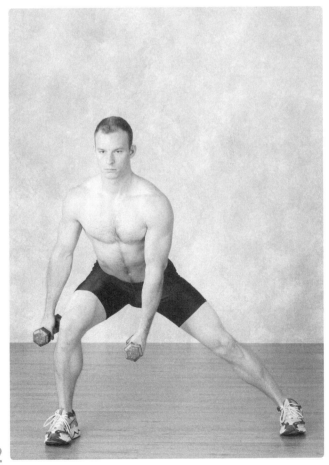

2

Rotation Lunge With Dumbbells

This works your whole lower body at the same time. By doing lunges along the transverse plane, rotating as you step, you work your external hip rotators. These muscles attach in and around the bottom of your pelvis, contributing to the integrity of your pelvis and pelvic floor.

Stand with your feet hip-width apart, holding a dumbbell in each hand (1). Turn to the left and lunge with your left leg toward a spot behind you, as if stepping to 7 o'clock on the imaginary clock described in the previous exercise (2). Return to the starting position. Now turn in the other direction and lunge with your right leg to where number 5 would be on your clock.

As a variation, you can do a clock lunge that mixes lateral lunges and rotation lunges. To do this, you step into a lateral lunge to 3 o'clock with your right leg, then step back to center; do a rotation lunge to 5 o'clock with your right leg, then step back to center; switch to your left leg and step to 7 o'clock, then step back to center; and finally step into a lateral lunge to 9 o'clock with your left leg. You can then repeat the clock in a counterclockwise pattern.

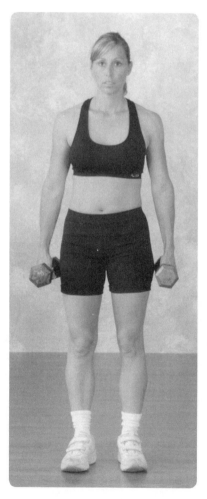

1

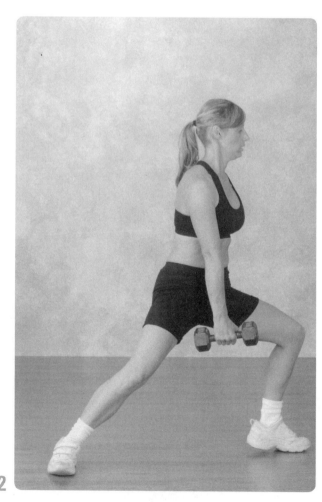

2

Jump Lunge

This exercise works all the parts of your lower body together, deriving much of its challenge from the jumping. Stand in a lunge position, with your feet about hip-width apart, both pointing straight ahead, and a stride length of about two feet (.6 meter). The length of your stride is correct when your knees form right angles as you bend them. Put your hands on your hips, lunge down slightly toward the floor (1), and then jump up with your entire body (2) and land softly.

You should observe that your knees are not collapsing in very much as you land. If your knees do cave in, include more of the single-leg squats in your workouts to get stronger in each leg. You should also do the band walking exercise described later in this chapter. Your landings should also be relatively quiet, which shows you that your body is absorbing the force well and not putting too much strain on your joints. When you finish your repetitions on one side, switch to the other.

If you can do one jump lunge and hold your position for two or three seconds after you land without collapsing or losing your balance, then you can progress to three to five repetitions in a row. Once you are able to perform more than five repetitions in a row with good form, you can try to do the jump lunges a tiny bit deeper, but again, do only three to five to begin with. This is an important principle of safe progression—when you increase the difficulty by making the lunges deeper, you should reduce the number of repetitions until you can do the deeper ones in good form. Then you can continue to progress, doing up to eight repetitions, although the more repetitions you do, the harder it will be to do them very deeply.

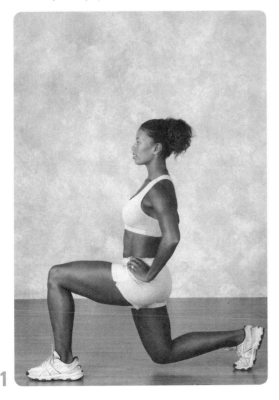
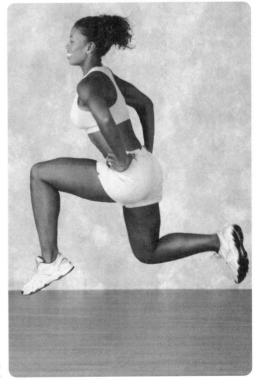

Step-Up With Dumbbells

Step-ups work your whole lower body at once, as well as create impact, which is good for challenging the integrity of your joints. When doing step-ups, you should start with a relatively low surface to step up onto, such as the platform of a step or a curb outdoors. The more you do this exercise, the higher you can make the step. The way to judge whether a given height is appropriate for you is to see if you can stay fairly stable in your midsection as you perform the exercise, without needing to hike your hip up as you lift your leg.

Get a step or a sturdy box about 8 to 12 inches (around 20 to 30 centimeters) high. Stand facing the step, holding the dumbbells at your sides. Step up with your right foot (1), then your left (2). Make sure you step onto the box with the entire surface of your foot. Step down with the right foot, then the left. After one set, start the next set with the left foot first. Step quietly and softly, staying strong in your core.

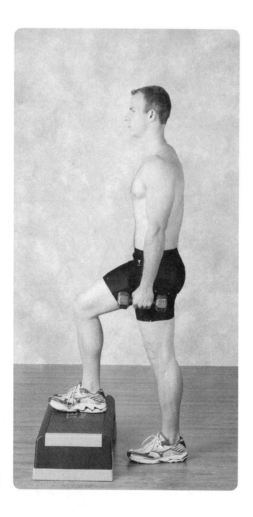

1

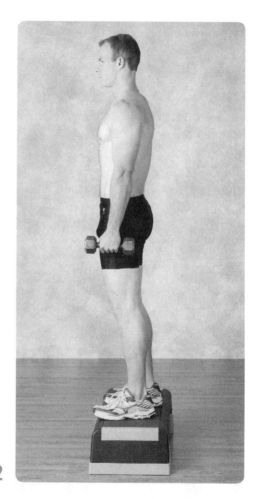

2

Deadlift With Barbell

This works your hamstrings and glutes and challenges your low back to stabilize the movement. Doing deadlifts is a great way to teach yourself how to move from your hips instead of from your spine. To get a feeling for the movement before you begin, stand with your right side facing a mirror. Keeping your knees straight but unlocked, lean forward from your hips. You should see that the slight curve in your low back does not change as you lean forward.

Stand with your feet pointing straight ahead, hip-width apart, and keep your knees straight and stable, but not locked. Hold the barbell down in front of your body, keeping your arms straight, with one hand in an overhand grip and the other hand in an underhand grip (1). Maintaining a neutral spine, lean forward from your hips (2). Only lean as far as you can keep the natural curve in your low back—you shouldn't see any change in the curve in your low back as you lean forward. Exhale as you stand up tall.

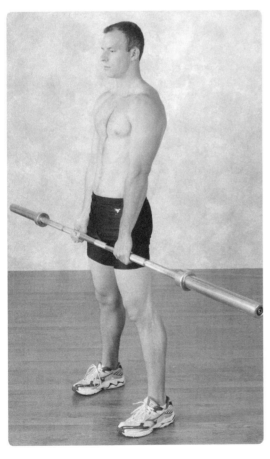

1

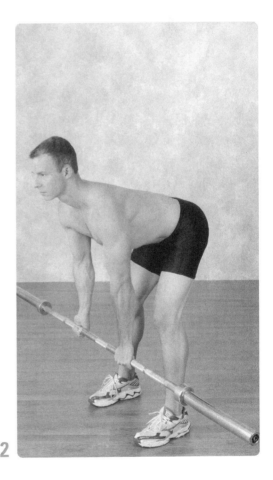

2

Bridge With Lower Body on Stability Ball

This exercise works the muscles around your hips, including the gluteus maximus, medius, and minimus. It also challenges your adductors and your core, which has to work to keep your body stable as you do the movement.

Lie on your back. Put your legs on the ball and straighten them out. The bigger the ball, the harder this exercise becomes. Start with the backs of your calves on the ball. As you get better at the exercise, you can place the ball farther down your lower legs toward your ankles. Lay your arms out to the sides so that your body forms a letter T (1). Maintaining a neutral spine, lift your hips off the floor (2). Try to do the exercise without pushing your arms into the floor or straining your neck. As the exercise gets easier for you, you can bring your arms closer to your body.

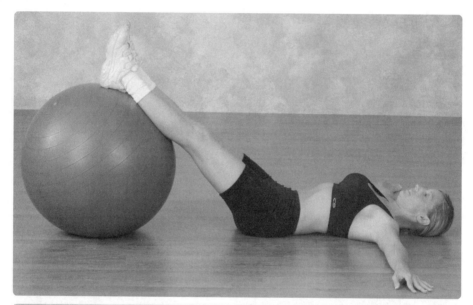

1

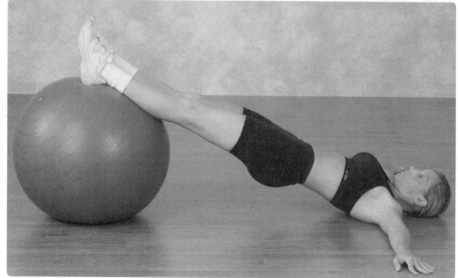

2

Bridge With Upper Body on Stability Ball

Like the previous exercise, this challenges all the muscles around your hips, but here you will also have to balance your body on the ball, which increases the demand on your core. Choose a ball that is big enough so that your thighs are parallel to the floor when you sit down on it.

Start by sitting tall on the ball. Walk forward, lying down onto the ball as you do so. Keep going until your shoulders and head are on the ball, with your neck neutral. Place your feet hip-width apart, and your knees at 90 degrees. Put your hands either on your hips or cross them over your chest (1). Without losing your neutral spine, lower your hips about halfway to the floor (2). Push them back up again as you exhale.

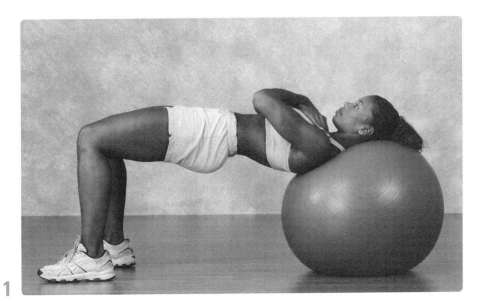

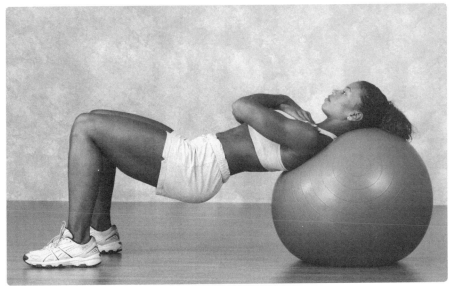

Single-Leg Bridge on Floor

This is a great exercise for the gluteus maximus and the other muscles around your hip (such as the gluteus medius and minimus), as well as your adductors and your core. Lie on your back with your knees bent and your feet on the floor, hip-width apart. Lift up your left foot and hold it up (1). Maintaining neutral spine, exhale as you lift your hips up in the air (2). Lift them high enough to get your body in a straight line from your chest to your knees.

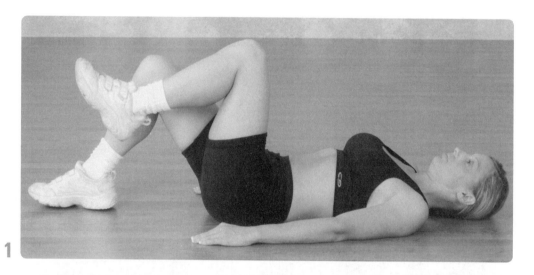

1

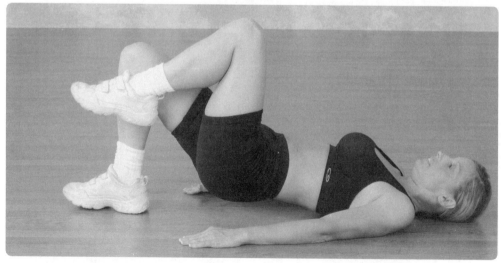

2

Band Walking

This is a great exercise to target the gluteus medius muscle of your outer hip. As mentioned in chapter 4, many times the gluteus medius is weaker than it should be. Isolating this muscle is a great idea if you notice the compensations discussed in chapter 4, such as your thighs collapsing in easily or your foot flattening out too much and continuing on up the chain of your entire leg.

Get a circular piece of tubing, or tie the ends of a piece of tubing together to form a loop. The circle should be small enough that when you step into it and stand with your legs about hip-width apart, you can already feel the tension. Put the tubing around your lower legs, above your ankles. If you see your knees caving in as you do this exercise, then put the tubing higher, above your knees around your thighs. Keep your knees soft. Put your hands on your hips and walk 10 steps to the left, then return. Keep your hip bones still as you walk, not letting them hike up as you step to the side. If you feel it is difficult to keep your hip bones still, lessen the tension in the tubing or take smaller steps.

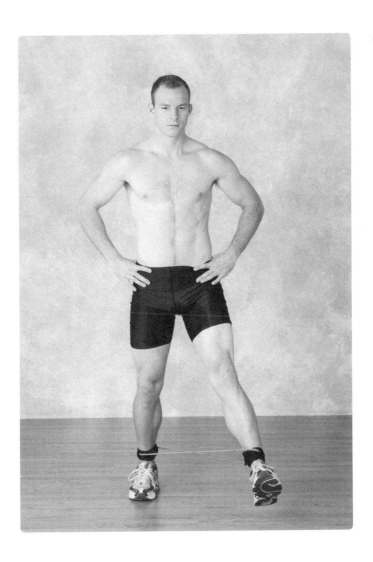

Single-Leg Heel Raise With Dumbbell

This exercise works your calf muscles (i.e., the gastrocnemius and the soleus). Stand on an elevated surface with your heels hanging off the edge. Hold a dumbbell in your left hand, and if necessary, use your right hand to hold on to something so you can keep your balance. Put your feet right next to each other, and then lift up your left foot, keeping it close to the right one (1). Lift your right heel up and down (2). When you have finished your repetitions, switch sides.

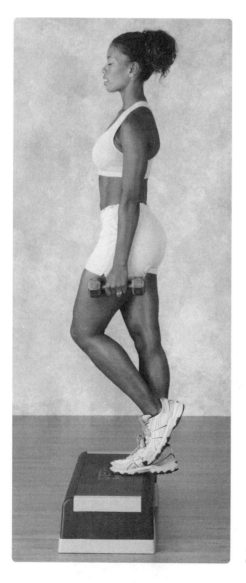

1

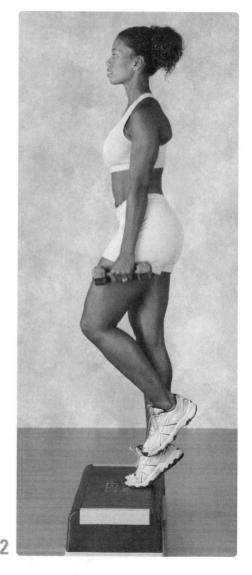

2

Single-Leg Heel Raise With Foot Turned In With Dumbbell

Traditional heel raises are done with the feet pointing straight ahead, but in this version you will turn your foot in to target the tibialis posterior muscle along with the gastrocnemius and soleus. Your tibialis posterior is a deep muscle that runs behind your tibia, or shinbone, and underneath your foot to help support your arch. As mentioned in chapter 4, if your arches tend to collapse inward, you should do this exercise regularly to keep this muscle strong. By turning your foot inward you are inverting it, which is what the tibialis posterior does, along with helping the other calf muscles to plantar-flex your ankle.

Stand on an elevated surface with your heels hanging off the edge. Hold a dumbbell in your right hand, and if necessary, use your left hand to hold on to something so you can keep your balance. Put your feet right next to each other, and then lift up your right foot, keeping it close to the left one. Turn your left foot in, keeping it flat with your toes turning in toward the right (1), and lift your left heel up and down (2). When you have finished your repetitions, switch sides.

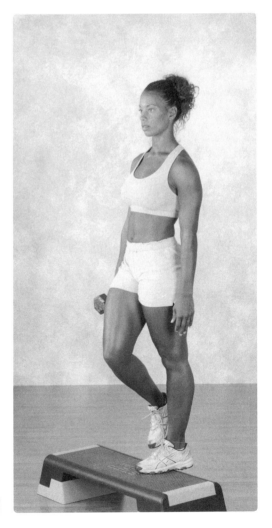

1

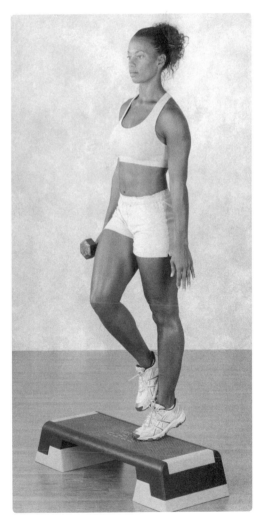

2

Leg Press

This exercise works your whole lower body at the same time, particularly challenging your quadriceps. There are many kinds of leg-press machines to be found in gyms. Some of them work by the seat moving; others work by the platform moving away from you as you push. The explanation of this exercise is based on the latter kind, but the seat setup will be basically the same on any leg-press machine.

When you perform leg presses, it's important to keep your feet pointing straight ahead and hip-width apart. Keep your neck neutral—your chin should not be too far forward. Sit on the chair of the leg-press machine and put your feet on the platform. Adjust the seat so that you can start with your thighs fairly close to your body, but you are still able to keep your neutral spine as you lower the weight, without your butt curling under. Position your feet on the platform so you start with a right angle at your knees, and keep your feet hip-width apart (1). As you exhale, straighten out your knees and push the platform away. Keep pushing until your knees are straight (2). Allow the platform to come back to the starting position without letting your butt curl under.

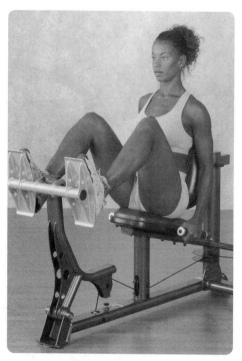
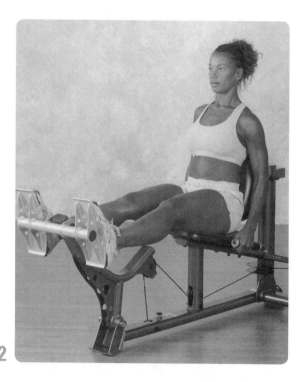

1

2

Single-Leg Press

As you perform the exercise, be sure to keep your neck neutral—your chin should not be too far forward. Sit on the chair of the leg press, and put your feet on the platform. Adjust the seat so you can start with your thighs fairly close to your body but are still able to keep your neutral spine, without your butt curling under, as you lower the weight. Put your feet on the platform so you start with a right angle at the knees, keeping them right next to each other. Lift up your left foot and hold it about three inches (seven or eight centimeters) off the platform (1). As you exhale, straighten out your right leg and push the platform away with your right leg (2). Your left leg should not move as you do the exercise with your right leg. Keep pushing out until your knee is straight. Then allow the platform to come back to the starting position, without letting your butt curl under. Keep your hip bones still throughout the movement. When you have finished your repetitions, switch to the left leg.

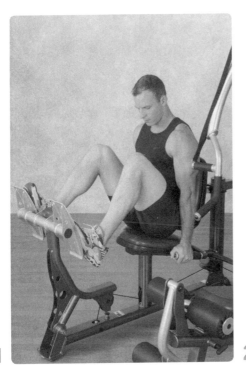

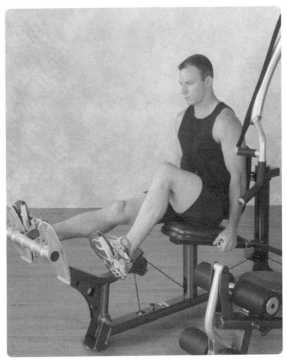

Leg Extension

This targets your quadriceps, the four muscles of the front of your thigh. In contrast to the squats and lunges earlier in the chapter that work various parts of the lower body at the same time, this exercise really isolates the muscle group. Adjust your seat position by lining up the rotation axis on the machine (right off the front of the machine seat) with your knee, right behind your patella, or kneecap. The pad at your shin should be a few inches above your ankle. You can tell it's in the correct position when it does not move up and down along your shin as you do the exercise.

Sit up tall on the machine pad (1). Exhale and straighten out your legs at the knees (2). Bring your legs back to the starting position.

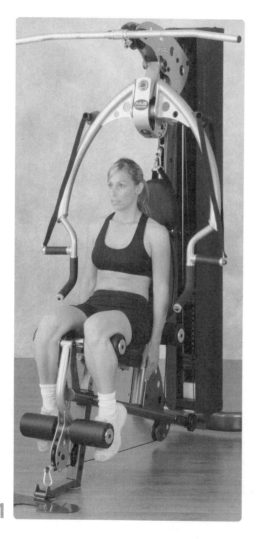

1

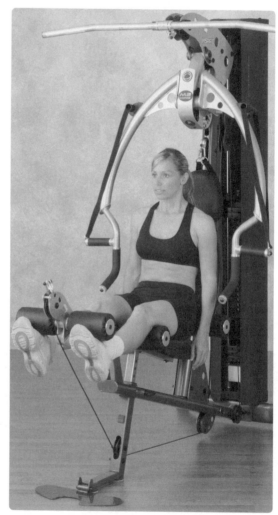

2

Index

Note: Figures are indicated with an italicized *f.*

About the Author

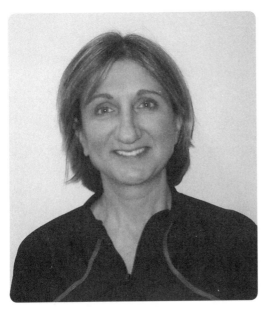

Annette Lang has been a Reebok University instructor since 1996, developing education programs for both fitness professionals and consumers. She is a regular consultant for NY Sports, Crunch Fitness, NY Health & Racquet, Bally Total Fitness, Wellbridge, and Equinox fitness clubs. She is a featured speaker at national fitness conventions, including the IHRSA International Conference and IDEA World Fitness Convention. She offers instruction and online courses through www.ptonthenet.com. Since 2000, Lang has served as a judge for *Fitness Management* magazine's Fitness Business NOVA awards for health clubs. Lang also worked with Peter Greenberg, the travel editor of NBC's Today Show, on his exercise and diet program. Her exercise program and motivational encouragement are also featured in Greenberg's book *The Traveler's Diet* (Villard 2006). Lang also wrote the *Prenatal & Postpartum Training Fan* (Benefit Health Media, 2006). She is certified as a personal trainer through the National Academy of Sports Medicine (NASM), National Strength and Conditioning Association (NSCA), and American Council on Exercise (ACE), and she has a master's degree in health education. Lang resides in Brooklyn, New York, and does private personal training in New York City. For more information, visit www.annettelang.com.

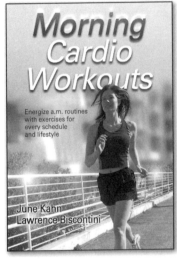
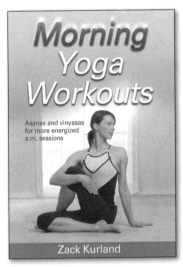
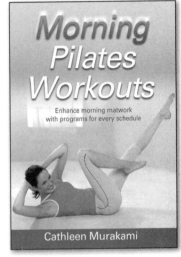

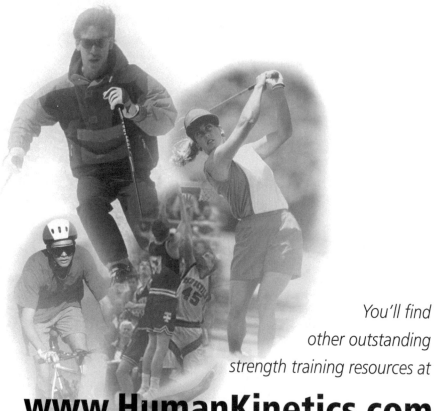